Joseph Joal, Richard Norris Wolfenden

On Respiration in Singing

Joseph Joal, Richard Norris Wolfenden

On Respiration in Singing

ISBN/EAN: 9783337182472

Printed in Europe, USA, Canada, Australia, Japan

Cover: Foto ©Andreas Hilbeck / pixelio.de

More available books at **www.hansebooks.com**

ON RESPIRATION
IN SINGING.

BY

DR. JOAL

(OF MONT DORE).

TRANSLATED AND EDITED BY

R. NORRIS WOLFENDEN,

M.D., CANTAB.,

FOUNDER (WITH MORELL MACKENZIE) AND EDITOR OF
"THE JOURNAL OF LARYNGOLOGY, RHINOLOGY,
AND OTOLOGY,"

*Late Senior Physician to the Hospital for Diseases of the Throat
Golden Square; and Vice-President of the British Laryngo-
logical Association; Fellow of the American Laryngo-
logical Association, and of the French
Society of Laryngology; Consulting
Physician to the Pearl Life
Assurance Company,
etc.*

𝔍llustrated with 𝔠oloured 𝔣rontispiece, and a number
of 𝔇iagrams in the 𝔗ext.

𝔏ondon:

F. J. REBMAN,

11, ADAM STREET, STRAND.
1895.

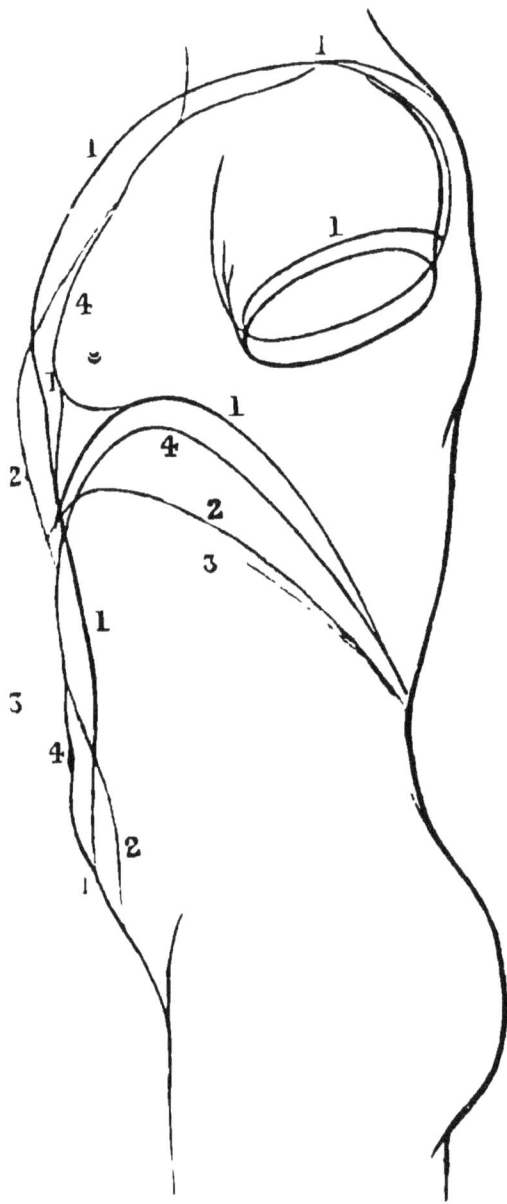

Fig. 1.—Diagram showing the three types of respiration.

1. Clavicular respiration.
2. Costal   ,,
3. Abdominal   ,,
4. { Outline of thorax and abdomen }
   {   before inspiration.   }

TRANSLATOR'S PREFACE.

I HAVE translated this little book, written by my friend Dr. Joal, because I think it contains useful information which may be laid to heart by the embryo singer. I do not believe that the art of breathing properly is sufficiently well taught to the singing pupil. In fact, my experience as a musical amateur, and as a physician practising the specialty of laryngology, is, that, in this country at least, the pupil is too often left to evolve a method of respiration from his or her own inner consciousness, and that singing masters very often pay no heed to what is the foundation of successful effort—namely, a correct method of breathing ; and, when they do endeavour to inculcate instruction in the art of breathing properly, each possesses a method of his own, sometimes founded upon a superficial and incorrect acquaintance with anatomy and physiology, generally a repetition of some phrases relating to the diaphragm, the abdominal muscles, etc., which they have had taught to them in their student days, and which they have imperfectly comprehended. It is no reproach to singers that they should know little about the anatomy or physiology of the respiratory organs ; but those who teach should have at least an elementary knowledge of these matters, otherwise their instruction is founded upon unintelligible data. What was the wise teaching of the old Italian masters no present-day teacher seems to know. Yet Gottfried Weber, " one of the most acute investigators who has studied the science of singing, says that it is impossible to explain why it is so, but that undoubtedly the old Italian method is the best."* The well-known maestro, Lamperti, is supposed to have inherited the traditions of the old Italian masters ; yet, on the other hand, the professors of the abdominal method have laid claim to him as one of their brethren. So far as we have been able to learn from those

* *Cæcilia* (1835), vol. xvii., p. 260, quoted by Morell Mackenzie, *Hygiene of the Vocal Organs*, 1st edition (1886), p. 109.

who may claim to have known something of his methods of instruction, we have always supposed him to have been strongly opposed to the "abdominal method" of breathing. Dr. Holbrook Curtis, in a paper recently contributed to the *New York Medical Journal* (Jan. 20th, 1894), remarks: "Having treated many of the elder Lamperti's pupils, and interrogated them very particularly upon this question, I may unhesitatingly affirm that the elder Lamperti was a strong advocate of the lower costal respiration, always arguing that the abdominal wall should remain quiet, or be slightly drawn in during inspiration. The evidence of Campanini, Jean de Reszke, and Clara Heyen is in support of the foregoing." Dr. Curtis's paper is one which will well bear perusal by both singers and teachers, and his conclusions are in agreement with the teachings of this little book—teachings which, consisting in inculcating thoracic respiration by raising the ribs and drawing in the abdomen, were the principles enunciated by such eminent teachers as Manuel Garcia, Mannstein, Carulli, etc. With the onslaught of Mandl upon the methods of the Paris Conservatoire commenced a new era of teaching; and this

b

author's ideas have more or less completely dominated the instruction of those singing masters who give any attention to the subject ever since. Attention has been largely directed to the method of " abdominal breathing," and the whole efforts of the pupil have, so far as breathing is concerned, been concentrated upon " descent of the diaphragm." Whether this quite modern method is any improvement upon the older doctrine it is the object of this book to show. It certainly possesses no advantages to the singer, in giving him a greater degree of inflation of the lungs. Happily, the tortures which were at one time imposed upon the pupil, in order to enable him to accomplish the control of this " descent of the diaphragm," are no longer practised ; but young singers are often even still put through unnatural, so-called " physiological," exercises to attain this end.

Mr. Lennox Browne, who has hitherto been generally known as a strong advocate of the views of Mandl,* has latterly entered the lists in severe opposition to Dr. Joal.†

---

* Morell Mackenzie, *loc. cit.*, p. 108. See also Curtis (*New York Medical Journal*, Jan. 20th, 1894).

† *The Medical Week*, vol. i., No. 41, Oct. 13th, 1893.

"Were it not," says he, "that the great work of Mandl, in insisting on the importance of inspiration for voice use being effected primarily by contraction of the diaphragm, *had been recently disputed* I would not do more than make bare allusion to this point ; for it really seems absurd that a muscle such as the diaphragm, which from earliest infancy is the sole one used for inflating the lungs in sleep and for the ordinary breathing purposes of life, should be ignored or treated as secondary to the action of the intercostal muscles, which take no part in filling the bases of the lungs—in other words, in deep breathing— so necessary for a full air-blast ; and yet, such is the fact.

" The only thing to be said in excuse for this new line of thought is that it is a reaction against the overswinging of the pendulum by Mandl. . . .

" Joal, on the other hand, and supporting him Wolfenden, contend that, so far from permitting a convexity of the epigastrium, the result of diaphragmatic contraction, they would have a concavity such as one would see in paralysis of that muscle, a lesion not only fatal to voice, but also to life." This is a misrepresentation of what Dr. Joal does really say or what his translator has ever said. I may refer to Chapter IX. of this little book, and to the diagram upon p. 111, to refute Mr. Lennox Browne's statement. It is not, however, my intention to enter into an argument upon the statements and mis-statements of the preceding lines of Mr. Lennox Browne's or of other portions of his recent paper. At a meeting of the British Laryngological Association* this author's collaborator (Mr. Behnke) spoke as if the descent of the diaphragm was the "be all and end all" of respiration for singing purposes,† and we took occasion to strongly dissent from such a view. It would seem, however, that there is not such a serious difference of opinion between Browne himself and Joal, as the remarks of the former would lead us to suppose, since he is credited in the French translation of his work with recognising that correct inspiration leads to " the increase in volume of the lower part of the chest and the upper region of the abdomen. The swelling of the abdomen ought to be limited to the

* 1892.
† *Journal of Laryngology,* June 1892.

epigastric region, and ought not to extend to the hypogastric region"; a considerable modification of the views as to "diaphragmatic" respiration which every one has been accustomed to attribute to Messrs. Browne and Behnke. There is, then, no question of attributing to the one author a statement that the singer should breathe with a "concave" abdomen, or to the other that he should breathe with a "convex" abdomen. Since Mr. Lennox Browne appears, in his later writings, inclined to share the views of both the author and translator of this book as to the correct aspect of the abdomen and dilatation of the lower part of the chest in breathing, we must attribute Mr. Lennox Browne's hypercritical remarks rather to a natural literary pugnacity than to the expression of any serious difference of opinion.

Some authors have seemed to imply by their writings that if there be not "abdominal breathing," there must of necessity be "clavicular breathing," ignoring the fact that there may be employed a third method, viz., what is sometimes called "costal breathing," the advantages of which it is the purpose of this book to support. The employment of "costal breathing" by no means implies any such error as "clavicular breathing."

But it is not my desire here to advance arguments or criticisms of the one method or the other. Dr. Joal's monograph deals fully with these matters, and must speak for itself. I have preferred to translate it as literally as is compatible with the exigencies of our own language, and to preserve the form of Dr. Joal's book as much as possible. If some phrases strike the reader as Gallicisms, he will attribute it to a desire upon the part of the translator to allow Dr. Joal to speak for himself and not merely through the mouth of a second person. I have added a few notes here and there, where it has been thought desirable.

Few authors sit down nowadays to write without imagining that they are going to "supply a long-felt want." Neither author nor translator arrogate to themselves this proud consciousness, but the latter thoroughly believes that in presenting this little work in an English garb he is doing a service to hundreds of amateur and professional singers, by directing their attention to principles which are the foundation of their art, viz.,

the use of their breathing organs in a rational
and effective manner. There would be fewer
broken voices and injured careers, fewer
patients for the laryngologist, if these principles were laid to heart by the singer and
even by the public speaker, for there is no
manner of doubt that an incorrect method
of breathing has more to do with vocal failures
and the production and aggravation of throat
troubles in the singer than any mere local
conditions.

I believe that this little book ought to be
in the hands of every one who aspires to sing,
and it is precisely because I think it to be
a valuable work, by a man who is both an
accomplished musical amateur, the intimate
friend of celebrated artists, and also an accomplished physician, that I have presented
it to English readers. The diction has been
purposely chosen to suit the intelligence of
lay readers, as distinguished from the medical
public. Finally, I little doubt that my fellow-
physicians will find much in this book to
interest them. A knowledge of the correct
method of breathing for the singer is, I feel
constrained to say, very much to be desired,
even among throat specialists, and much more

among singing masters. In these days of Board Schools, it is imperative that more and greater scientific attention should be paid to this subject. We are called upon almost daily to treat young women whose vocal organs have failed, through the efforts of continuous teaching—speaking and singing— which they are called upon to exert. Too many and continuous hours of work, classes too large for the efforts of one individual— and that nearly always a young person in the early years of puberty—classrooms hot, stuffy, and dusty, all contribute to the end, viz., the breakdown of the voice of the young teacher. I have myself seen so many cases of this character, that the occurrence of frequent voice failure in young Board School teachers cannot be regarded as accidental. Indeed, I cannot but think that the work thrown upon these young persons sometimes makes the Board School teaching system a public scandal, and one which certainly de- mands open medical inquiry and readjustment. Proper voice training might undoubtedly remedy the defect very considerably, and this training should have for its foundation a proper and scientific teaching of the art of respiration both for public speaking and singing. Without advocating this or that method, it is highly desirable that an official scheme of instruction should be adopted— and one such could easily be formulated by a committee of laryngologists and singers— and this scheme should be the basis of instruction in every board, and public, and private school in the Kingdom. Surely it is a subject important enough, for it embraces the care of the youth of the country, many of whom in after life become public speakers, orators, teachers, and singers, to begin the serious labours of life handicapped by an imperfect knowledge of the manner in which to use their vocal organs, and too often to break down prematurely, from the abuse of these organs, which early and proper training would have avoided.

R. NORRIS WOLFENDEN

35, HARLEY STREET, W.

CONTENTS.

TRANSLATOR'S PREFACE . . . . pp. vii—xvi

INTRODUCTION . . . . p. I

CHAPTER I.

THE RESPIRATORY ACT. ANATOMY AND PHYSIOLOGY.

The thorax ; its form ; bones which compose it. Bronchi,
lungs, pleural cavity.—Inspiration : elevation of the
ribs, external inspiratory muscles, diaphragm.—
Expiration : *rôle* of the thoracic walls, passive in
simple, active in forced, expiration . . pp. 4—14

CHAPTER II.

RESPIRATORY TYPES.

Clavicular, abdominal, and costal types : their definition.
—In ordinary respiration the child employs the
abdominal method ; the adult man sometimes the
abdominal, sometimes the costal, method.—The
woman uses the clavicular method.—Influence of
corsets.—Pneumographic tracings of non-civilised
women.—Preponderance of the action of the diaphragm in tranquil respiration . . pp. 15—23

xx CONTENTS.

CHAPTER III.

ORDINARY AND ARTISTIC RESPIRATION.

Aim of ordinary respiration ; aim of artistic respiration :
the latter necessitates deep inspirations, which require the intervention of thoracic muscles. Opinion
of physiologists.—Great development of the chest
in gymnasts and singers.—The play of the
thorax is the principal factor of respiration in
singing . . . . pp. 24—34

CHAPTER IV.

HISTORY OF ARTISTIC RESPIRATION.

Teachings of the old Italian masters, and of the authors
of the old method of the Conservatoire.—School
of Mandl.—The old practices are abandoned.—
Triumph of abdominal respiration . pp. 35—45

CHAPTER V.

CLAVICULAR RESPIRATION.

It has the inconvenience of being partial, amplify-
ing the thorax at the summit of the cone, and
furnishing the singer with less wind than the two
other types.—It has not the disastrous effects attributed to it.—Refutation of Mandl's ideas as to
lowering of the larynx, glottic dilatation, relaxation
of the cords as the consequence of this defective
practice.—Clavicular respiration cannot be recommended to man or woman, although the latter
breathes with the summit of the chest in ordinary
life . . . . pp. 46—61

CHAPTER VI.

ABDOMINAL RESPIRATION.

It permits the storing of a greater volume of air than clavicular respiration ; but it only utilises the contraction of the diaphragm, and leaves the thoracic muscles inactive.—Whatever the method of respiration, muscular fatigue is in direct relation to the effect produced ; it is manifested less quickly when the work is divided between a large number of agents.—Why has nature given us a mobile thorax, if it ought to remain in a condition of fixity in the deep respirations needed for singing ?—Abdominal respiration submits the stomach, uterus, and other viscera, to strong pressure. Morbid accidents in consequence . . . . . . pp. 62—78

CHAPTER VII.

COSTAL RESPIRATION.

The movement of dilatation is general, and the chest participates as a whole in the inspiratory amplification.—The thorax is enlarged in its greatest diameter, the transverse.—Geometrical formula relating to the valuation of the thoracic volume.—Spirometric researches prove that it is the costal method which provides the greatest amount of air for the singer . . . . pp. 79—90

CHAPTER VIII.

COSTAL RESPIRATION (*continued*).

The artist can regulate the exit of air with precision.—
Vocal effort, muscular antagonism, and synergy.—
Insufficiency of abdominal force.—Respiratory
mechanism of the *mezza di voce*.—On thoracic
resonance ; the sonorous properties of the pectoral
cavity are brought into play by the costal
type . . . . pp. 91—109

CHAPTER IX.

COSTAL RESPIRATION (*continued*).

Movements of the ribs in costal respiration.—*Rôle* of the
diaphragm.—Doctrines of Magendie, Duchenne,
Paul Bert.—Retraction of the abdominal wall,
limited to its inferior portion, favours elevation of
the ribs by the diaphragm.—The old Italian masters'
advised the costal type.—Professors and physicians
who recommend this respiratory process, and artists
who practise it . . . . . pp. 110—130

CHAPTER X.

EDUCATION OF RESPIRATION.

Importance of good respiration in singing.—Characters
of inspiration and expiration in an experienced artist.
—Necessity of beginning respiratory studies early.—
Methodical exercises applied to costal respiration. —
Duration of the exercises ; avoidance of fatigue.—
Ordinary gymnastics augment the respiratory
power . . . . pp. 131 147

CHAPTER XI.

HYGIENE OF RESPIRATION.

Necessity of good hygiene.—Influence of vitiated, humid, dry air.—Action of dust : nasal inspiration.—Dwellings : apartments, heating and lighting.—Clothing : flannel, corsets, braces, belts.—Food : nitrogenous and carbonaceous ; spirits, coffee.—Hours of repose. —Muscular exercise . . . . pp. 148—168

CHAPTER XII.

RELATION OF THE MOTOR TO THE VIBRATING ELEMENT OF PHONATION.

Height of a sound.—Aerial pressure in laryngeal intonation.—Agreement between the muscular agents of respiration and the larynx.—Vocal compensation.— Respiratory insufficiency robs the voice of its freshness, purity, agility, and extent.—Laryngeal fluxions, acute and chronic laryngitis . . . pp. 169—183

CHAPTER XIII.

ETIOLOGICAL CONDITIONS CAUSING LOWERING OF THE VITAL CAPACITY.

Utility of spirometric measurements.—Respiratory feebleness due to change of method.—Nasal affections : obstruction, reflex phenomena.—Hypertrophy of the palatine and lingual tonsils ; chronic pharyngitis. —Onset of emphysema and pulmonary tuberculosis. Gastralgias, flatulent dyspepsias.—Gaseous distension of the intestine . . . . pp. 184—198

APPENDIX.

The resonance of the thorax.—The influence of odours and perfumes upon the voice.—Local conditions leading to impairment of the voice.—Laryngitis in singers.—Cocaine .   .   .   .   . pp. 199—208

INTRODUCTION.

THE subject which we are about to study is not concerned exclusively with physiology ; it has an artistic side, the importance of which cannot be misconceived. We should never, however, have ventured to write this book if we had not been able to supplement our scientific acquirements with some vocal and musical knowledge, and, moreover, if we had not been able to apply ourselves personally to the art of singing.

For a long time we have been occupied with the interesting question : how is it necessary to breathe for singing ? At the commencement of our medical career, more than twenty years ago, we were greatly impressed by reading the famous memoir of Dr. Mandl, and our personal experience has since placed

I

us in opposition to the doctrine of abdominal respiration. But it then seemed to us rash to take part in favour of the old Italian method, and to combat the new doctrines accepted in France by most professors of singing.

Our opposition was quite Platonic until 1885, an epoch when we had the good fortune to enter into relationship with M. Jean de Reszke, who, himself an ardent partisan of costal respiration, persuaded us to break a lance for the good cause. This illustrious artist has never ceased to give us his excellent advice, and has permitted us to put under great contribution his large experience and remarkable erudition in the art of singing ; and we are glad to recognise this by dedicating this book to him.

We lean upon the indisputable authority of M. Jean de Reszke in recommending singers to take their breath according to the following rules :—

1. Not to raise the clavicles or the upper ribs.

2. To fully dilate the lower portion of the thorax.

3. To depress the abdominal wall in its

lower portion, about the umbilical and hypo-gastric regions.

We shall begin by recalling some anato-mical and physiological ideas necessary to the comprehension of the subject. We shall study the different respiratory types, showing the inconveniences and the advantages of each method, and establishing the superiority of the costal type over the clavicular and ab-dominal. Then we shall glance at artistic respiration from the points of view of its education and hygiene. Lastly, having in-dicated the vocal troubles engendered by respiratory feebleness, we shall add some words upon the morbid states which diminish the pulmonary capacity. Our aim will be obtained if we succeed in convincing our laryngological *confrères*, professors of singing, and artists, of the justice of our ideas, and if we are able to lead them back to the wise traditions of the old Italian masters.

CHAPTER I.

THE RESPIRATORY ACT. ANATOMY AND PHYSIOLOGY.

The Thorax: its form; bones which constitute it, bronchi, lungs, pleural cavity.—Inspiration: elevation of the ribs, external inspiratory muscles, diaphragm.—Expiration: function of the thoracic wall, quiet in simple expiration, active in forced expiration.

THE apparatus of phonation is composed (1) of the nasal fossæ, the mouth, the pharynx, a vocal tube which modifies and re-enforces the sound; (2) of the larynx, of which the inferior cords produce the sound, vibrating under the influence of the current of the expired air; (3) of the trachea and bronchi, which constitute a veritable *porte-vent*; (4) of the thorax and lungs, which have a double function, viz., that of furnishing the air and that of re-enforcing the sound; their action is comparable to that of the bellows of the organ, and at the same time

4

to that of the sounding board of the piano.
We have no need here to occupy ourselves
with the upper portions of the human instrument—the nose, mouth, pharynx, and larynx.
We shall limit ourselves to stating some
elementary anatomical and physiological ideas
concerning the constitution and the function
of the respiratory bellows, which alone in-
terests us at this moment.

If we examine the chest of a well-consti-
tuted individual, it presents the form of a
quadrangular pyramid, the base of which is
formed by the shoulders, and the summit of
which is lost in the abdomen.

But this chest, deprived of its soft parts
and of its muscular masses, is of quite
different aspect : the thoracic cage then represents a cone slightly flattened from before
backwards, the summit of which is at the
shoulders. The cone is limited, behind by
the dorsal portion of the vertebral column,
in front by the sternum and clavicles, and
laterally by the ribs, which, on the skeleton,
are separated from one another by spaces, but
which, on the living subject, are united by
the internal and external intercostal muscles,
thus making all these osseous arcs continuous

one with another. The base of the cone is formed by one large muscle, the diaphragm, which is attached entirely to the inferior edge

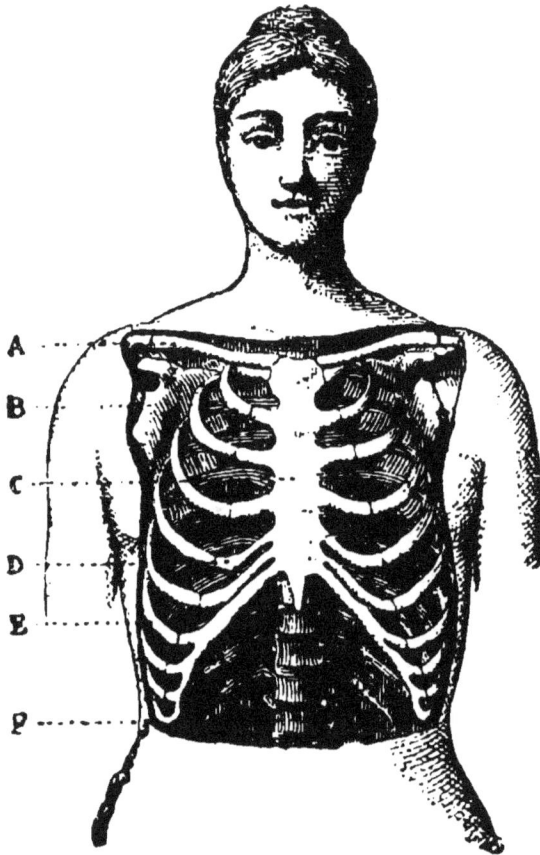

FIG. 2.

A. Clavicle.   D. Sterno-costal cartilages.
B. Scapula.   E. Sixth rib.
C. Sternum.   F. Vertebral column.

of the thorax, thus separating the thoracic from the abdominal cavity. The summit of the cone is entirely occupied by the organs which proceed from the neck to the thorax. Among these structures must be mentioned the tracheal tube, which puts the thoracic cavity, closed in every part, into communication with the atmospheric air. It is in this chamber with its osseo-muscular walls, and occupying the greater portion of it, that the lungs are lodged ; one portion of the cavity being reserved for the heart and great vessels. The lungs, completely separated from one another, and of different volume, have the form of a cone at the summit. Each of them is essentially constituted of numerous canals, which divide and subdivide to infinity, and successively bear the names of large, median, and small bronchi, and respiratory canaliculi. These last ramifications end in a *cul-de-sac*, a small cavity called the pulmonary lobule, and composed of the pulmonary vesiculi. These vesicles are like the leaves of the respiratory tree ; it is upon their surface that the gaseous exchanges are made between the blood and the atmospheric air.

It has been calculated that the lungs of an adult man contain not less than six hundred millions of these vesicles. Between the lungs and the thoracic walls exists a serous cavity, the pleural cavity, which, in its normal state, is entirely empty, containing neither water, gas, nor liquid. The two surfaces of the pleura can play and glide over one another; but they cannot be separated, since the atmospheric pressure which is exercised upon the internal surface of the lung maintains them applied one to the other.

The lung, according to Matthias Duval,* adheres to the thorax, and ought to follow each movement of it, just as a stone, to which has been exactly applied a piece of wet leather, follows the latter when it is raised. This well-known children's device represents the mechanism by which the thoracic cone forces the pulmonary cone to dilate at the moment of *inspiration*, the first act of respiration, which it is now necessary for us to study.

The inspiratory movement effects an increase in the capacity of the thoracic cage, separating the base from the summit, and the lateral walls from each other, or, as may be said, augmenting it in three diameters; the antero-posterior, transverse, and vertical dia-

* *Cours de Physiologie.*   Paris : Baillière.

meters of the thorax. The antero-posterior and transverse diameters are enlarged by one and the same movement, namely, the elevation of the ribs.

The ribs, which are osseous arches, obliquely directed from above downwards, from behind forwards, and from within outwards, are supported behind upon the vertebral column, which is immovable, and are united in front with the sternum, which is a movable point. It appears to us easy to understand that if the anterior extremities of the ribs are raised, the sternum is carried forward and must be separated from the vertebral column, thus enlarging the antero-posterior diameter of the thorax.

It is the same as in the case of the two uprights of a ladder with oblique steps ; when the uprights are separated from one another the steps approach the horizontal. Moreover, the inclined plane from within outwards, and from above downwards, which the rib forms, is raised, turning round an oblique axis, which passes from the sternum to the vertebral column, and which represents the chord of the arc formed by the rib ; the convexity of this is then carried outwards, and from

thence results the transverse dilatation of the
thorax. These movements of the ribs are
dependent upon the action of certain muscles
called the elevators of the ribs. These, in
ordinary inspiration, are : the external intercostals (levatores costarum), the scalenes, the
serratus posticus superior, and the cervicalis
ascendens. In more ample inspiration there
is super-added the action of the serratus
magnus, the pectoralis major, the pectoralis
minor, and the latissimus dorsi. Lastly, in
forced inspiration, there also come into play
the sterno-cleido-mastoidei, the trapezius, the
rhomboids, the levatores anguli scapulæ, the
splenius, the recti capitis antici major and
minor.

The lengthening of the vertical diameter
is due to the contraction of the diaphragm.
This large muscular septum is inserted behind
to the lumbar vertebra by two large muscular
bundles, having a vertical direction, and called
the pillars of the diaphragm, upon the six
last ribs, and anteriorly, to the point of
the sternum. All the fibres issuing from
these points of insertion converge towards a
common centre, aponeurotic, and having the
shape of a trefoil leaf, and called the phrenic

centre.* The surface of the diaphragm is much more extensive than the circle formed by its points of insertion, which presents the aspect of a vault with a convexity upwards, upon which rest the heart and neighbouring parts. It is generally supposed that this muscle straightens its curvature upon its contraction, and that it then augments the vertical diameter of the cavity of which it forms the base, the latter being convex towr.ds the upper part during the repose of .ie muscle, and almost plane during its cor raction. But we shall remark, '+h M .:ias Duval, that the curvature of ..phragm is exactly moulded upon that o1 r. ¯ 1ial viscera, to the right, for exampic, ..;on that of the liver ; therefore, when the muscle is contracted, it can only feebly modify this convexity or curvature, which it displaces rather from above downwards, pushing before it the viscera. It therefore acts after the fashion of a piston of convex form, which moves in the body of the pump represented by the thoracic cavity.

We shall see further on that to this action

* Called by English anatomists the " central or cordiform tendon of the diaphragm."—ED.

of the diaphragm upon the vertical diameter of the chest there is added a second, and more disputable, action upon the other diameters.

The arched centre of the muscle would then become comparatively fixed, taking support from the abdominal viscera ; and its periphery, of which the points of costal insertion are movable, would be carried upwards, from whence arises elevation of the ribs, and, secondly, increase of the transverse and antero-posterior diameters. In a word, during inspiration the dilatation of the thorax is effected in every sense, and it is produced by the intervention of muscular power. The lungs are here purely passive, the active *rôle* belonging entirely to the thoracic cage.

In expiration, which constitutes the second period of the respiratory act (expulsion of air), the active *rôle* is reserved to the lungs, the thoracic walls becoming in turn passive. The pulmonary organ is indeed contractile and elastic.

Its contractility is due to the presence of smooth muscular fibres (muscles of Reisscissen) in the walls of the small bronchi. Elasticity is a property which the pulmonary tissue possesses in the highest degree, and which is easily demonstrated in the following manner :—

The respiratory organs of a calf having been obtained from the butcher, the lung is insufflated through the windpipe. It is dilated by the air, but returns suddenly upon itself, immediately insufflation ceases. It acts, in fact, like a caoutchouc ball. From this the mechanism of expiration will be easily explained.

At the moment of inspiration the lungs accompany the movements of the thoracic wall only in spite of themselves, their elasticity struggling against the inspiratory muscles. But when these muscles cease to contract, and immediately the pulmonary elasticity, the play of which is no longer impeded, regains its liberty of action, the lungs return on themselves, and, owing to the pleural vacuum, draw with them the thoracic walls. Expiration is thus effected in the ordinary conditions of life.

On the contrary, in forced expiration the thoracic walls do not merely follow the movement of the retreat of the lungs ; they assume an active *rôle*, and compress the lungs, augmenting the speed and energy of the current of air. Certain muscles then come into play, and act in a sense inverse to the inspiratory forces, lowering the ribs. These inspiratory muscles are the internal intercostals, the infra-costals, the triangular muscle of the sternum, the serratus posticus inferior, the quadratus lumborum, and the muscles of the abdominal wall in certain conditions. We shall see that, in singing, expiration is always active.

CHAPTER II.

RESPIRATORY TYPES.

Clavicular, abdominal, costal types: their definition.
—In ordinary respiration the child adopts the
abdominal method; the adult· man sometimes
uses the abdominal method, sometimes the costal.
—The female employs the clavicular method.—
Influence of the corset.—Pneumographic tracings
obtained from non-civilised women.—Preponderance of the action of the diaphragm in tranquil
respiration.

I N the ordinary movements of respiration
the enlargement of the chest does not
equally affect the three diameters of the
thorax. In different individuals dilatation is
effected in different ways by the thoracic walls,
occurring either over the upper region, the
median portion, or the base of the chest. It
is sufficient, in fact, to glance‾at some persons
to state that some breathe with the abdomen,
others with the chest.

The method of inspiration can be varied

experimentally. By strongly compressing the thorax in its inferior portion, the enlargement of the chest is effected particularly at the expense of its upper portion.

If the thoracic enlargement is principally manifested in the region of the upper ribs, the respiration is called *clavicular*.

In the *costal* type the respiratory movement is especially marked over the region of the median and inferior ribs.

In the *abdominal* type the enlargement of the chest results chiefly from the action of the diaphragm.

Most authors admit these three respiratory methods ; for example, Beau and Maissiat,* who in 1842 first gave an excellent description, from which we quote the distinctive characters as follows :—

"**Clavicular type.**—The greatest extent of movement is over the upper ribs, and especially the superior, which are carried upwards and forwards. The clavicle and the sternum participate in this movement, which diminishes as we descend from the superior to the inferior ribs. The abdomen is drawn in during inspiration.

* *Archives générales de Médecine,* 1842-43.

"**Abdominal type.**—In this method there is nearly complete fixation of the thorax. The movement is made by the abdomen especially over its median aspect. The diaphragm contracts, taking a point of assistance from the ribs. The phrenic centre is lowered and the abdominal viscera are pressed downwards, pushing forward the abdominal wall during inspiration.

"**Costal type.**—The changes occur especially over the inferior ribs. The sternum moves downwards, while its upper portion remains immovable, like the first rib. The abdominal wall is not pushed forward as in inspiration, and, in certain subjects, it is even flattened."

In ordinary calm and tranquil respiration, individuals, then, make use of one of these three types. It is interesting to seek what physiological conditions may influence the inspiratory method.

Numerous observations and repeated experiments have proved that the method of inspiration varies according to the age and sex of the subject. Authors are unanimous in maintaining that the child uses the abdominal type. But as to the adult man there is a divergence of opinion. The majority of

physiologists profess an opinion which is
generally accepted in the scientific and artistic
world ; to wit, that man employs the abdominal
type. On the contrary, Dally, Witkonski,
Bergonié, and Viault attribute to man the
employment of the inferior costal type. These
latter authors * thus express themselves in
their recent work, the result of researches
undertaken by means of the graphic method
—that is to say, with registering instruments :—

" If there are applied successively in a man,
a woman, and a child, three identical pneumographs, placed on the body at different
heights, the first surrounding the chest at
the level of the upper ribs, the second at the
level of the inferior ribs, the third at the level
of the umbilicus, it can be demonstrated
that the curves traced by the three pneumographs have very different amplitudes on
the same subject, and vary even with the
subject.

" In a man respiring calmly, the first pneumograph, at the level of the upper ribs, inscribes only feeble amplitudes ; the second,
at the level of the inferior ribs, inscribes

* *Traité de Physiologie humoine.* Paris, 1884 : Doin.

amplitudes comparatively greater ; the third inscribes intermediary amplitudes. The inspiratory movement is then effected especially at the level of the inferior ribs.

" In a woman it is otherwise ; the amplitudes inscribed by the upper pneumograph surpass all the others.

" Lastly, in the child it is the pneumograph round the umbilicus which furnishes the greatest amplitude."

Which of these two opinions ought we to adopt ? Does man breathe, in the normal state, by the abdomen or by the inferior part of the thorax ? In order to determine this point we have examined a large number of subjects, and, with Longet, Küss, and Matthias Duval, we adopt the opinion of Beau and Maissiat, who wrote in their remarkable memoir in the *Archives Générales de Médecine* : " According as individuals advance in age, there is observed the predominance of the superior costal type in the feminine sex, and *the nearly equal proportion of the other types in the masculine sex.*" That we believe to be the truth.

As to the *female*, we have just seen, by the two preceding quotations, that she respires

with the upper region of the chest, and that
she expands particularly the upper ribs.   All
agree in recognising this fact.

Mandl,* however, takes exception to this,
and writes : " It is an error to believe that
the clavicular type is natural to women.   On
the contrary, it never exists in the normal
condition. . . . The   natural   type,   if   it   is
not abdominal, is lateral."

To what physiological condition can we
attribute the difference of the respiratory
method in the two sexes ?

According to some authors it is because
clavicular respiration is the only method which
does not impede the genital functions of the
female ; in fact, during pregnancy, the diaphragm cannot, without inconvenience, fully
contract and press upon the gravid uterus.

These physiologists remark that this method
of respiration constitutes a true sexual characteristic, since Haller and Bœrhaave have stated
its occurrence in little girls one year of age.
Bérard, Longet, Hutchinson, Küss, and Duval,
accept this view.   Other scientists, and amongst
them Beau and Maissiat, Walshe, Sibson, and
Regnard, incriminate, on the contrary, the

* De la fatigue de la voix.   Paris, 1855 : Ed. Labbé.

constrictive action of the corset; but the influence of this article of clothing was never demonstrated. To-day, however, the problem appears to have been determined, thanks to the researches undertaken during recent times by two American physicians.

Dr. Mays * (of Philadelphia) has studied by the graphic method the respiratory movements of eighty-two girls of from 10 to 22 years of age, belonging to an uncivilised race. Thirty-three of these girls were Indians of pure breed; thirty-five were half-breeds. In all these subjects an abdominal and a costal tracing were taken. Seventy-five times out of eighty-two the pneumograph revealed a method of respiration purely abdominal. The girls exhibiting the costal type were found to come from tribes comparatively civilised, such as the Mohawks and Chippawas. A Michigan *confrère*, Dr. Kellog, made similar researches upon forty women, of whom twenty were Chinese and twenty Indians, and the registering instruments always demonstrated the abdominal method. This physician has, moreover, examined a certain number of women of the Cherokee and Chukassaw tribes.

* *Journal of Physiology*, March 1890. Cambridge.

Those who wore corsets respired with the chest, and others who were not so compressed with clothing breathed by the abdomen. From these facts the direct intervention of the corset appears no longer to be doubtful. Consequently it is natural to attribute to the same influence the development of the clavicular type in young girls of our country.

The continual use of the corset, worn during nearly three hundred years by many generations, has led to modifications of the respiration, at first temporary. These have been transmitted by heredity, and have ended in constituting what Hunter and Darwin call a *secondary sexual characteristic*—that is to say, a character which has no immediate relation to the act of reproduction.

If we put on one side the respiratory method of the woman, which is vitiated by the use of the corset, it results from the preceding physiological facts relative to the man and child, that in ordinary tranquil respiration the movements of amplification are observed at the base of the thorax, that the increase of volume of the chest occurs principally in the vertical and tranverse diameters, enlarged especially by the contraction of the diaphragm.

Certain authors even consider this muscle to be the inspiratory muscle almost exclusively, and maintain that it alone acts in the abdominal and inferior costal types. In the first case, the lowering of the diaphragm is pronounced, the compressed viscera are pushed downwards and forwards, producing extrusion of the abdomen. In the second case the descent of the muscle is less marked ; the *phrenic centre* maintained by the liver, the stomach and the spleen, becomes a fixed point of contraction ; it is the peripheral insertions which are movable, and which, projected outwards, determine the elevation of the ribs.

According to the individual subject the abdominal wall is then immovable in inspiration, or is slightly flattened. We think that the *external inspiratory agents*—that is to say, the muscles of the thoracic wall—intervene to raise the inferior ribs when, in the inferior costal type, we observe flattening and retreat of the abdominal wall.

However that may be, we do not hesitate to recognise that the diaphragm plays a preponderating *rôle* in the mechanical phenomena of ordinary respiration,

CHAPTER III.

ORDINARY RESPIRATION AND ARTISTIC RESPIRATION.

The aim of ordinary respiration and of artistic respiration; the latter necessitates deep inspirations, which require the intervention of the thoracic muscles. Opinion of physiologists upon this point.—The great development of the chest in gymnasts and in singers.

THE play of the thoracic cage is the principal act of respiration in singing, from the fact that, in ordinary respiration, movement of the ribs does not constitute the most important factor of thoracic dilatation, and from the fact that the work of the external inspiratory muscles is relegated to a secondary place. Certain physicians and professors of singing have deduced an argument in favour of the abdominal method which they recommend to artists.

Respire naturally, say without cessation to their pupils these masters who repel as unphysiological every inspiration not

characterised by swelling of the abdomen.
It, however, appears to us (1) That the act
of respiring to oxygenate and purify the
blood is not the same as the act of breathing for singing ; (2) That the mechanism
of simple, tranquil respiration differs from
the mechanism of complex respiration with
effort.

In *ordinary respiration* we introduce atmospheric air into the chest. This air penetrates
into the pulmonary vesiculi, of which the walls,
excessively thin, are clothed with a very fine
network of small capillary vessels. It is
there that the gaseous exchange is produced
between the blood and the air necessary for
life ; the blood absorbs fresh oxygen and
throws off carbonic acid in excess, which
could not remain in the organisation without
poisoning it. Each respiratory movement
causes the entry of a small quantity of air,
on an average half a litre, into the pulmonary
cavity. These movements are repeated fifteen
times a minute ; that is to say, they have a
medium duration of four seconds for inspiration and expiration, the former being a little
shorter than the latter. By the effect of
inspiratory dilatation the intrapulmonary

pressure descends to 99·5 (the external pressure being represented by 100).

This pressure mounts to 100·5 during expiration.

In *artistic respiration* it is necessary, on the contrary, (1) To make an ample provision of air ; (2) To drive it out under strong pressure ; (3) To manage and regulate the exit of the breath ; (4) To increase the resonance of the thoracic cavity.   It is also necessary to have at disposal a pretty considerable quantity of air, often surpassing $3\frac{1}{2}$ litres.   We have even observed more than 5 litres, by the aid of the spirometer.

The second phase of the respiratory move-ment is characterised by its longer duration. Sounds are very frequently held more than twenty seconds.   We have noted even forty.

During inspiration the intra-pulmonary pressure is easily reduced to 90.

During expiration it is not rare for this pressure to rise above 115.

These numbers, expressing the volume, the exit, the pressure, of the air in artistic respira-tion, differ sensibly from those which we have indicated previously for ordinary respiration.

A simple glance at these figures shows that,

in singing, new muscular forces must be brought into play ; (1) in order to augment the capacity of the chest ; (2) in order, when the thoracic walls are widely dilated, to retard their retraction by regulating the exit.

In a word, the respiratory mechanism employed for the habitual needs of life is insufficient for the singer, who cannot content himself with the isolated action of the diaphragm, and who must utilise all the muscular powers destined for *ample, exaggerated, complex,* and *forced respiration.*

Authors employ these different denominations to qualify, according to the amount of the amplification, great respiratory movements.

But almost all physiologists agree in recognising that, in deep respirations, the *rôle* of the diaphragm is not so preponderating, and that of the costal apparatus largely aids the thoracic dilatation. " In exaggerated inspiration," say Beau and Maissiat,* " there is seen in the same individual a combined movement, which results from the union of two types, and sometimes even three."

Berard† writes also : " In calm respiration

* Memoir already quoted.
† *Traité de Physiologie.*

many subjects seem to respire only by the diaphragm and with a very slight movement of the ribs. In exaggerated respiration everything comes into action ; the diaphragm, movement and rotation of the ribs, and an elevating movement of the ribs and the sternum."

According to Béclard,* " when a person respires very deeply, all diameters of the chest are simultaneously increased, and the movements of the ribs and the movements of the diaphragm are carried to their utmost limits."

According to Sibson,† " when a person respires as deeply as possible, the movements of the ribs and the diaphragm are more accentuated than in calm respiration, but the augmentation of that of the ribs is most pronounced."

We read in Wundt : ‡ " In tranquil and normal inspiration, the pressure exercised by the diaphragm causes the upper portion of the abdomen to project ; in very deep inspiration,

* *Traité de Physiologie.*
† *Med. Chirurg. Transactions*, t. xxxi.
‡ *Physiologie humaine*, French translation by Bouchard.

on the contrary, the diaphragm being obliged to follow the ascent of the ribs, the same region of the abdomen is slightly depressed."

Viault* emits the opinion "that, in the case of forced inspiration, there is no longer any great difference between the two principal respiratory types, superior costal and inferior costal, as in calm respiration. The displacement of the sternum becomes considerable in this case, and it is in the region of the first ribs that the thorax presents its maximum dilatation." And, among the physicians who have occupied themselves with the vocal art, Charles Bataille † writes : " In the normal condition, when a person is lying on the back, and the respiratory rhythm is abandoned to itself, the movement of elevation of the ribs, almost imperceptible over the upper portion of the chest, becomes more and more pronounced as we descend, and the abdomen is largely pushed forward by each inspiration. On the contrary, when the movement of inspiration is exaggerated, the superior costal respiration assumes a considerable development."

* *Traité de Physiologie.*
† *De l'enseignement du chant.* Paris, 1863 : Masson.

Morell Mackenzie * also remarks, in speaking of the deep respirations necessitated by great efforts, " that the abdominal walls are depressed in inspiration. The diver who is going to plunge into the water, the warrior who is about to deliver a mighty blow instinctively draws in and fixes the abdominal walls." And, lastly, Sewal † affirms that the type is always costal when the respiratory needs of man are urgent.

The importance of the point to be established justifies the numerous quotations which precede.

It would appear to us, therefore, indisputable that in deep respirations the dilatation of the chest ought to be effected in its three diameters, and that amplification ought to be total and not partial.

The researches undertaken by Marey ‡ upon the gymnasts of the Joinville school give support to this conjecture, and demonstrate the activity of the costal apparatus in exaggerated respirations, as, for instance, in

* *De l'hygiène des organes de la voix.* Paris : Dentu.

† *Journal of Physiology*, March 1890. Cambridge.

‡ *Comptes rendus Acad. des Sciences*, 1880.

running.   This eminent experimenter, having
chosen five young pupils, took, with the
pneumograph, tracings of the respiration ;
firstly during repose, then after a race of
six hundred mètres,* and showed that in the
latter case there was a notable amplification
of the chest.   The same experiment was
repeated many times.

After a month, the amplitude of the thoracic
movements during repose had more than
doubled ; at the end of five months, it
had more than quadrupled, and it was
then impossible to remark any respiratory amplification under the influence of
racing.

Chassagne and Dally† have also made
studies upon the soldiers of the Joinville
school.   They have measured the chests of
these young subjects at the time of their
entering the school.   After five months of
training the measuring was repeated, and, in
307 gymnasts out of 401, it was found that
the bi-mammary thoracic circumference had
sensibly increased.

* About 700 yards.
† *Influence précise de la gymnastique sur le dévelop-
pement de la poitrine.*   Paris, 1881.

Morell Mackenzie * also relates that " Maclaren, so long the Mentor of the athletic youth of Oxford, says that the effect of walking exercise has often been shown in his own person by the gain of some inches of chest girth in the course of a short pedestrian excursion."

À priori, the singer ought to profit by the same advantages as the runner; exercise ought to increase the proportions of his chest. This is, indeed, what observation shows.

We have often been agreeably surprised to see what beautiful forms and what a superb aspect the upper portion of the thorax has presented in our artists of renown.

Segond had before made the same remark.†
" Singing," said he, " by increasing the activity of the organs of respiration, soon determines their growth ; and most singers present a great development of the thorax." Dally ‡ said the same ; " in singers we find, as in those statues which represent typical beauty in the highest degree, a chest sensibly convex,

* *Loc. cit.*
† *Hygiène du chanteur.* Paris, 1846 : Labbé.
‡ *Bulletin général de thérapeutique,* 1881.

surpassing by many centimètres the shoulder measurement."

This increase in the antero-posterior and transverse diameters can evidently only be attributed to the exercise, and to the supplementary work which is effected in the different parts of the thorax and in the muscles which are inserted there.

From all these facts, it results that physiological laws command the singer not to breathe *only* with the diaphragm, but also, and *especially*, with the external dilating muscles of the thorax.

We shall show further on that in practice inspiration ought not to be pushed to excess; the first ribs and the clavicle remaining motionless, the amplification of the chest should attain its maximum at the level of the seventh rib, and the base of the thorax. The abdominal wall is depressed in its two inferior thirds. Lastly, we remark that, in artistic respiration, during expiration the inspiratory muscles continue to contract and struggle against the expiratory agents in order to oppose a too rapid reduction of the diameters of the chest.

These phenomena of struggle and opposition between the different forces are no other than those described by authors under the name of *effort*.

According to the happy definition of Ledentu,* effort is a sum total of intense muscular contractions having for a condition the complete or incomplete fixation, general or partial, of the thorax, with or without suspension of respiration.

In another part of this work we shall maintain that the act of singing is of the variety described by Verneuil † under the name of *thoracic effort*. We will here be content with remarking that there cannot be any fixation of the thorax without previous dilatation of the costal apparatus, and without contraction of the elevating muscles of the ribs.

This physiological theory furnishes us again with an argument in support of our thesis. *In singing, as in all deep respirations, the play of the thorax constitutes the principal factor in the enlargement of the chest.*

---

* Art. *Effort. Dictionnaire Méd. et Chir. pratiques.*
† *Société de Chirurgie.* Paris, 1836.

CHAPTER IV.

HISTORY OF ARTISTIC RESPIRATION.

Teachings of the old Italian masters, and of the authors of the old method of the Conservatoire.—School of Mandl.—The old practices are abandoned.— Triumph of abdominal respiration.

W E have seen that, in ordinary life, three respiratory methods are employed to renew the oxygen of the blood.

These types, although under the control of the will, and capable of modification by education, are those which are met with in a general manner in singers, in whom they are found, however, with characters less clear and distinct, in consequence of the amplitude of the respiratory movements.

Not to make any new classification, we will recall :—

    1. Clavicular respiration, viz., that in which, on inspiration, *the first ribs and the clavicle are raised, and the abdominal wall is strongly drawn in* ;

2. Costal respiration, viz., that in which, on inspiration, the upper ribs and clavicle being immovable, the enlargement of the chest is produced over the region of the *middle and lower ribs*, while the *abdominal wall is slightly depressed in its two inferior thirds* ;

3. Abdominal respiration, viz., that in which, on inspiration, there is *comparative fixity of the ribs, and protrusion of the abdomen.**

As is very often seen in matters of art, these three methods have had partisans and adversaries equally resolute, whose arguments and criticisms we shall have to discuss. But it is necessary to remark that we shall only occupy ourselves with authors citing original facts, without entering into the region of fable.

---

* A striking instance of the power of controlling these abdominal muscles and the descent of the diaphragm, was on one occasion exhibited to me by Mr. Hamilton, a late "orator" at Buffalo Bill's Show. Standing between the wall and an average-sized cottage piano, with his back to the wall, and abdomen against the piano, he was able, by the protrusion of his abdomen alone, to push the piano from him several inches! He was otherwise a powerful and very muscular man. [Translator.]

We must say that we have only comparative confidence in the greater number of writers who, in presenting a history of singing, relate the vocal processes of great singers. Often " the wish has been father to the thought," and they have accommodated their facts to their theories.

Let us quote an example well proving this, viz., that of Rubini. Massini * and his pupils proclaim that the celebrated tenor was the promoter of abdominal respiration. Bonheur † says, on the contrary, that this singer dilated the upper part of the chest. Walshe ‡ relates that he fractured the clavicle during a violent effort to reach a high " b " in a recitative from " The Talisman," of Pacini. And, lastly, Lablache § and Laget ‖ avow that, in spite of long and attentive observation, in the theatre, they were not able to distinguish how the illustrious singer breathed.

How can any opinion be arrived at after

* Delprat, *La question vocale.* Paris, 1885.
† *Essai critique de l'enseignement vocal actuel.* Paris, 1891.
‡ *Dramatic Singing.* London, 1881.
§ *Méthode complète du chant.* Paris.
‖ *Le chant et les chanteurs.* Paris: Heugel.

such discordant statements? It is just the same as regards professors of singing. The famous Lamperti, of Milan is, turn by turn by different authors, represented as an upholder or adversary of the abdominal method, or yet again, as being indifferent as to the respiratory method.

As concerns artists, we shall content ourselves with quoting those whose breathing we have ourselves observed, generally in our consulting-room, or at least outside the theatre ; for, on the stage, it is not always easy to determine if it is the thorax or the abdomen which is most employed in inspiration.

This much being said, to show how difficult it is to expose the history of the subject, we must say further, that the old authors furnish us with but little documentary evidence concerning the point which occupies us.

" However well they may have understood the importance of respiration," say Lemaire and Lavoix,* " and whatever care, in their schools, the old Italian masters took to teach their pupils to respire properly, they have left us few positive directions on the subject."

* *Le Chant.*   Paris, 1881 : Heugel.

Tosi * limits himself to saying " the master ought to teach the pupil to direct his respiration well, to take in a little more than is necessary, but never in such a manner as to fatigue the chest. Mannstein † has, however, transmitted to us the method of the famous Bernacchi of Bologna (1775), who gives the following wise advice : " Inspiration ought to be produced without shocks and without protruding the abdomen. It is only the chest which should be raised. Inspiration ought to consist in absorbing rather than swallowing or gulping at the air. The better the singer can economise his breath, the less need has he of air in the larynx to form a full and round sound.

" That is why we recommend the following rules to him : the abdomen is protruded during respiration in speaking ; in respiration during singing it ought to be drawn in. In speaking the chest rises and falls suddenly ; in singing it ought to be raised and lowered insensibly, so that the air absorbed may suffice for a longer time."

* *L'Art du chant*, French translation by Lemaire.
† *Système de la grande méthode de Bernacchi, de Bologne;* Leipzig, 1835.

The Abbé Blanchet (1756) in his *Principes Philosophiques du Chant*, and Rameau (1760), in his *Code de Musique Pratique*, *à propos* of respiration, content themselves with some generalities, without entering into technical details.

It was at the commencement of the century that the *Première Méthode du Conservatoire* was edited by a committee formed by Cherubini, Méhul, Gossec, Garat, Guingéné, and the illustrious singer, Mengozzi.

In this work we find the excellent precepts of Bernacchi thus formulated :—

" The act of respiring for singing differs in some fashion from respiration for speaking.

" When we breathe for speaking, or simply to renew the air in the lungs, the first movement is that of aspiration, then the abdomen swells, and its upper portion advances a little ; then it relaxes ; that is the second movement, viz., that of expiration. These two movements occur slowly when the body is in its natural condition.

" On the contrary, in the act of respiring for singing, it is necessary, in aspiring, to flatten the abdomen and to cause it to return with promptitude, while swelling out, and advancing the chest. In expiration, the abdomen ought to return very slowly to its natural position, and the chest ought to be lowered, in order to retain the air which has been introduced, in the lungs for as long as possible. It should be allowed to escape only slowly, and, without giving any shocks to the chest, it should, so to say, flow out."

These counsels were generally adopted in our country, when, in 1855, there appeared in the *Gazette Médicale* the famous memoir of Dr. Mandl, advocating abdominal respiration.

"The deplorable doctrine of the Conservatoire," said this author, "can without hesitation be considered to be the cause of the loss of a great number of voices. To flatten the abdomen is to impede the normal lowering of the diaphragm, and to force the respiration to become clavicular when it is deep. We cannot, therefore, raise our voices with sufficient force to combat a fatal principle, especially when we see it figuring in an official method."

Mandl was not the originator of the abdominal system, but its eloquent defender and indefatigable populariser ; he, indeed, declared that his attention had been drawn to this type of respiration by Masset, who had himself seen it practised in Italy.*   One of the first promoters of the abdominal method in France was also M. Delsarte, who, since 1839, had taught it in his public classes.

Abroad Signor Massini appears to have been the great apostle of the new doctrines; we call them new because we do not meet with any trace of them in the writings of the old Italian masters, and we think that it is necessary to discover at all costs the claims to nobility of the abdominal method, in order to uphold the statement of Lemaire and Lavoix, that it was recommended by Blanchet and by Rameau.

However that may be, the ideas of Mandl were greeted with enthusiasm.

A veritable revolution was then accomplished in the teaching of singing.   Minds were impressed by the anatomical and physiological considerations which served as a foundation for the attacks made against costal respiration.   Professors, with a few exceptions, took upon themselves to destroy all that which they had previously adored; they forgot the judicious recommendations of Bernacchi,

* Memoir quoted.

and of Mengozzi, and taught only to breathe *diaphragmatically, abdominally, ventrally*; some of them even inventing for this purpose instruments of torture.

Certain vocal classes resembled, as Gustave Bertrand remarked,* cells of Charenton.   In order to immobilise the thorax, pupils were made to sing while lying down on mattresses, sometimes with weights, more or less heavy, placed on the sternal region ; masters were even said to make a practice of seating themselves familiarly upon the chests of their pupils.   In the schools were to be seen gallows with thongs and rings for binding the upper half of the body, orthopædic apparatus, rigid corsets, kinds of pillories which enclosed the frame, and immobilised the ribs. Oscar Comettant † relates that he had known a professor who reduced the whole art of singing to the following exercise : he placed a gag, a kind of *poire d'angoisse*, in the mouth of the pupil, and made him emit sounds which resembled a hiccough, obliging him to withdraw the diaphragm at each sound.   This

* *De la réforme des études de chant au Conservatoire.* Paris, 1871 : Heugel, éditeur.
† *Musique et Musiciens.*   Paris, 1862.

is the pleasant side of the campaign led by
the enthusiasts of abdominal respiration.

That which is more serious still is the fact
that the efforts of Mandl were crowned with
success ; he had, indeed, the sweet satisfaction
of seeing his system hall-marked by official
authority.

And in a new edition of the method of the
Conservatoire, published in 1866, by Batiste,
Mandl himself sang the praises of the abdominal type ; the chapter on *respiration* containing a note written by his own hand.

It is well to remark that the victory was
comparatively easy, enemies being somewhat
imaginary ; the artillery having been addressed against clavicular respiration, which
was not in the forefront of the battle. Mengozzi and his collaborators, indeed, only
recommended " the flattening of the abdomen,
and causing it to remount with promptitude
while swelling and advancing the chest."
They never spoke of raising the upper ribs
and the clavicle.

But flattening of the abdomen in no wise
implies the use of the clavicular type. We
shall see that Morell Mackenzie pronounced
himself against the employment of this latter

method, while advising depression of the abdominal walls during inspiration ; we shall defend the same opinion when, after having studied the clavicular and abdominal types, we shall estimate at their proper value the advantages of costal respiration.

CHAPTER V.

CLAVICULAR RESPIRATION.

This respiration has the inconvenience of being partial, by causing the thoracic amplifications to be carried out at the summit of the cone, and by furnishing the singer with less breath than the two other types.—But this respiratory method has not the disastrous effects which have been imputed to it. Refutation of Mandl's ideas on the lowering of the larynx, glottic dilatation, relaxation of the cords, which are said to be the consequences of this defective practice.—The use of clavicular respiration ought not to be recommended either among men or women, although the latter respire with the top of the chest during ordinary life.

THE clavicular type is a method of respiration of which the daily and continual employment cannot be recommended to singers.

In support of this opinion we will only point out one single consideration. Compared with the abdominal, and especially with the costal methods, the clavicular furnishes less air, since the thoracic dilatation is carried out principally at the summit of the respiratory cone, the point at which the diameters of the chest have the least extent.

The results which we have obtained with the spirometer put this fact beyond doubt : it is easy to convince oneself by glancing at the figures indicated further on (Chapter VII.).

But we must recognise that the discreet employment of the clavicular type, limited to the largest and deepest inspirations, as a complement to the costal method, has nothing reprehensible about it.

In any case, we cannot admit that this type of respiration is capable of producing all the evils of which it has been accused by Mandl.*

" We ought, before all," says this writer, " to banish from teaching and practice clavicular respiration, in which the vocal struggle and fatigue are very considerable.

" Indeed, many muscles which act during inspiration and expiration, from fixed and slightly flexible parts, are then displaced.

" The larynx is strongly lowered, the glottis enlarged, and the cords relaxed during inspi-

Fatigue de la voix (1855).

ration ; and, during expiration necessary to
the modulation of sound, these parts must

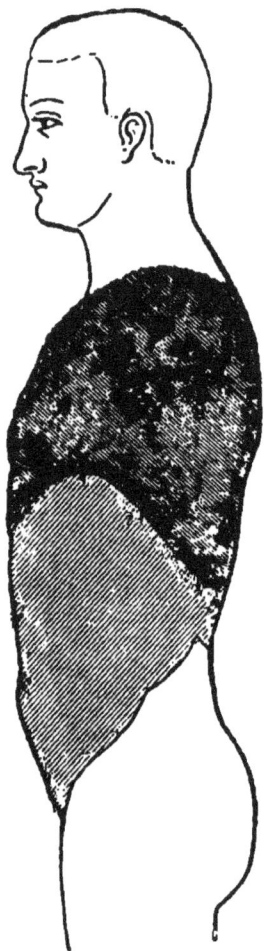

FIG. 3.
Side view of the thorax,
abdomen, and diaphragm
before inspiration.

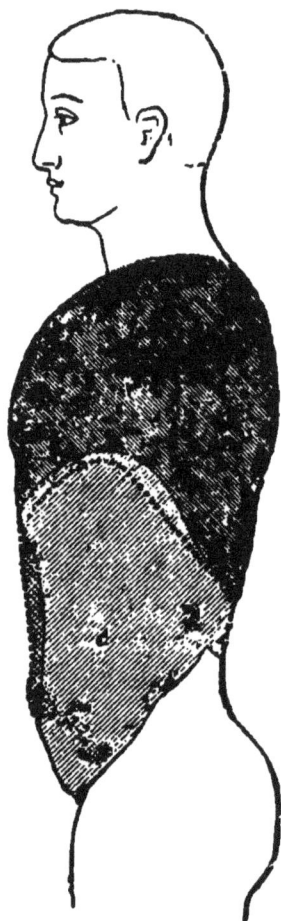

FIG. 4.
Clavicular type. The
dotted line represents
the side view before in-
spiration.

find themselves in conditions diametrically
opposed.

" All these movements are so interwoven the one with the other that the inspection alone of the clavicle allows one to define the position of the larynx. These opposite tractions, exercised upon the larynx during singing, when clavicular respiration has been adopted, render the emission of the voice more difficult, more fatiguing, and less harmonious."

And Mandl thus continues his description :—

" Considerable effort, swelling of the neck, enlargement of the jugular veins, throwing back of the head, and noisy inspiration, form the habitual accompaniment of this faulty respiration. It may even occasion at length in the muscles employed an excessive sensibility, and spasmodic contractions ; twitchings of the mammary region and sudden hoarseness are thus frequently explained. This pathological condition may in the intrinsic muscles of the larynx cause more or less complete atrophy, with loss of contractility and loss of voice consecutively."

Here, indeed, is a sombre picture, of a nature from its blackness to carry fright into the minds of artists who raise the clavicle in singing ; but they will be quickly reassured

if they read the book of M. Bonheur,* for
there they will learn that outside the superior
costal type there is no safety for voices, and
that the abdominal method is the most terrible
enemy of the singer.

"For a long time," said the Professor of
Liege, "there has been a wish to innovate
and to apply to the mass the respiratory
methods which can be employed only by a
few rare individualities—respiratory methods
approaching those of birds and quadrupeds,
whose particular structure forbids clavicular
respiration.

" I do not hesitate to declare that the decadence of the art of singing is due mostly to
the terrible errors which have crept into the
teaching of respiration, and which have been
propagated unhappily to such a degree that
they have almost become authoritative.

"It is to the dangers of these abnormal
methods of respiration, and principally of
abdominal respiration, that I wish to draw
attention. And I can do it with so much
more assurance, I may say even authority,

* *Essai critique de l'enseignement vocal actuel, avec
note médicale du* Dr. Cheval. Paris: Paul Dupont,
1891.

from the fact that I found my opinions upon my own experience, having myself been a victim of this fatal teaching."

Without accepting the ideas of Bonheur, we cannot sufficiently protest against the doctrine of Mandl, which is based upon false anatomical and physiological considerations, on imaginary ideas, and on facts badly observed or badly interpreted.

We do not speak for the present of fatigue of the thoracic muscles, which ought equally well to be manifested in the costal type, and with which we shall occupy ourselves later on ; but let us now refute the arguments based upon the pretended extrinsic and intrinsic movements of the larynx.

Is it true, as Mandl says, that while, in abdominal respiration, the larynx remains immovable, it is, on the contrary, necessarily lowered in the clavicular type during inspiration ?

We do not find this lowering mentioned in any of our classical treatises of physiology or anatomy, nor in any of the numerous works which have appeared since 1855 on laryngology, which leads us to suppose that other authors have not shared the ideas of Mandl upon this subject. And, moreover, we have examined in this respect a number of individuals whom we have engaged to breathe alternately by the abdomen and the shoulders ; and in ourselves we have often, while singing, observed the movements of our own larynx, and we have never been able to state that clavicular inspiration led, as a sequence, to the descent of the thyroid.

That which is true, and which is admitted by most authors, is that the larynx is lowered in all inspirations of a certain amplitude, and particularly in those which precede singing, whether the clavicle be or be not raised. Nicaise * has given us the explanation of this fact by the experimental demonstration that during deep inspirations the trachea is retracted, shortened, and draws down the larynx.

Another error of Mandl is in considering this lowering of the vocal organ to be produced by the necessary and obligatory action of the sterno-thyroid and sterno-hyoid muscles, which should contract with the scalenes, the sterno-mastoids, and other muscles, when these latter are required to raise the thorax, and

* *Revue de Médecine*, 1889.

which, inserted above on the hyoid and thyroid, which are movable points, and below upon the sternum and the first rib, which are fixed points, must approach their superior to their inferior insertions.

We do not think that the sterno-thyroids and sterno-hyoids are elevator muscles of the thorax; we do not believe in their community of action with the scalenes and sterno-mastoids. These latter receive their innervation from the cervical and brachial plexus, while the sterno-thyroids and sterno-hyoids are innervated by the descending branch of the great hypoglossal. These are scientific facts well established to-day, since the beautiful experiments of Wertheimer. This difference of innervation was unknown to Mandl; and it has the result of reducing to nothing the fundamental notions upon which he built his respiratory system.

And since we deny the lowering of the larynx, what must we say of the glottic dilatation and the considerable relaxation of the vocal cords which result from it, according to the same erroneous ideas, and which would have consequences so disastrous in the emission of the voice? Here we must remark that the work of Mandl dates from an epoch when laryngoscopy was not yet practised ; consequently all the glottic modifications of which he speaks are purely theoretical.

We ourselves have, on the contrary, often practised laryngoscopic examinations upon persons breathing with the summit of the chest, and we have never observed the phenomena in question. We therefore refuse to admit the famous laryngeal struggle (*lutte laryngée*) invented for the needs of his cause by the terrible adversary of the clavicular type. In this latter the larynx preserves a mobility as perfect as in the other respiratory methods.

For the rest, the principal professors of the abdominal school are not agreed even among themselves upon this point. Thus Ch. Bataille maintains that the glottis is retracted in place of being dilated, as Mandl pretends.

" When a person breathes," says Bataille,* " strongly and principally raising the upper ribs, the lips of the glottis, being energetically drawn towards one another by the violence

* *De l'enseignement du chant.* Paris, 1863 : Masson, éditeur,

of the current of air, leave between them only a very narrow space, and it is with trouble that the muscles of. the glottis succeed in maintaining the latter sufficiently open."

This divergence of opinion favours our views ; the respiratory method remains without influence upon the extrinsic and intrinsic movements of the larynx.

À propos of the frightful disorders indicated by Mandl as a consequence of clavicular respiration, we had already, in 1890, in a work entitled *Spirometic Researches in Nasal Affections*, emitted doubts as to the true origin of these symptomatic manifestations.

We have difficulty in believing, we said, that these accidents, and especially that dyspnœal crises, can be brought about by the employment of the clavicular method, since we see it every day in use among great artists and even in our most illustrious cantatrices. At the Mandl epoch there had been little pre-occupation with nasal affections, and reflex neuroses were not known. Can we not, moreover, defend the idea that certain of his patients, particularly those who had attacks of oppression, were individuals affected with respiratory troubles of spasmodic form and of nasal origin?

On the subject of the preceding lines, M. J. Weber, the learned and authoritative musical critic, has invited us* to cite some artists who employ the clavicular method with success. We should be very happy to comply with the wish of M. Weber, but it is very difficult for a physician to descend to personalities, and to say that such a singer employs a vocal process considered to be *disastrous* and *execrable* by the princes of criticism. In such a case one cannot have too much reserve and discretion. However, so as not to give the impression of retreating, we have obtained from our friend Melchissédec the authority to quote his example. This excellent baritone takes a breath by dilating the whole of his thorax and raising his upper ribs. For twenty-five years this eminent artist has been on the stage! Whoever has heard him sing during these later times is able to say that he is always in full possession of his vocal powers. The voice is always fresh, voluminous, well graduated, and very extensive; the sounds

can be held for more than forty seconds.
Lastly, there is not the least fatigue, not
the least susceptibility of the larynx : always
to the front at the Opera Comique, and at
the Opera, M. Melchissédec has been and
always is·the model of the *pensionnaires*, ready
to take his place at each representation.   We
can, moreover, affirm, from the aspect of the
glottis by the laryngoscope, that the use of
clavicular respiration has not been detri-
mental to him.

But let it not be concluded from this that
we counsel the superior costal type.   Quite
the contrary : we condemn its employment as
a general custom.

We content ourselves, in the face of the terrible accusations thrown against this method,
with pleading attenuating circumstances in
its favour, and with showing that it is not
responsible for the desolations and abomi-
nations attributed to it; for excellent artists
practise it and derive good results from it.

Just the same as regards abdominal
respiration.   We do not recommend it, but
we must recognise that it has been mar-
vellously utilised by singers of the greatest
value—MM. Obin and Faure, for example.

If we except the works of Laget* and Bonheur, we nowhere find the glorification of the clavicular type in man.

It is by design that we do not speak of the former method of the Conservatoire and the books of Mannstein, Carulli, and Manuel Garcia, because, in these treatises, there is contained no recommendation to raise the shoulders, but only to inspire by flattening the abdomen, and dilating the thorax by the elevation of the ribs, movements which, we shall see later on, are very well reconciled with absolute fixity of the clavicle.

MM. Dally and Cheval are, among physicians, those who have the most warmly pleaded the cause of superior costal respiration. The former, after having described and defined the three respiratory methods of Beau and Maissiat, says:—†

"We accept this analytical supposition rather as a method of study than as the expression of a physiological fact. In reality there is only one single respiratory type normal to man ; that is, the clavicular type, with this addition, that it excludes neither the

* *Le Chant et les Chanteurs.* Paris : Heugel, éditeur.
† *Bulletin général de Thérapeutique,* 1881.

movements of the inferior ribs nor that of the diaphragm. . . . But if we accept the precepts of some singing masters and of M. Mandl, we should encourage diaphragmatic respiration, to the detriment of costal respiration. It is total inspiration that it is necessary to teach."

Almost unanimously, then, authors condemn the clavicular type—at least, so far as it concerns man.

In the woman it is not so. A certain number of writers advise this kind of respiration, and among them our distinguished *confrère*, Dr. Hamonic.*

"Women," writes he, "breathe by the upper and very little by the inferior ribs. This difference is explained by the fact that if woman breathed like man, the uterus would be more or less compressed, and troubles would result during pregnancy. Those teachers, therefore, who make women breathe like men commit a physiological error. They go against nature, falsify it, and can only obtain bad results."

We ourselves do not agree with this opinion.

* *Manuel du Chanteur*. Paris, 1888: Fisbacher, éditeur.

We have already said that in the feminine
sex the employment of the clavicular type,
in ordinary respiration, was due to the use
of the corset, and that this practice was
vicious.

In singing, the woman ought to breathe
in the same manner as the man—that is to
say, to dilate everywhere the thoracic cage
in its middle and inferior parts, slightly retracting the abdominal wall below the sub-
costal line, and not raising the upper ribs.

Professors who enforce the adoption of the
costal type upon young girls act wisely.
With the least *maladresse* or indocility, the
clavicular method will, in general, be pretty
easily abandoned by young people who will
consent not to compress their figures.

On the contrary, in the case of non-success
it might be dangerous to desire to modify,
at all cost, the respiratory type. After fruit-
less trials, the prudent master will abandon
the effort, under pain of causing injury to
the freshness, the purity, the precision, and the
extent of the voice.

We may, in reference to this, cite the
unhappy example of a great artist to whom
had been promised the augmentation of the

power and volume of her voice. The implacable professor succeeded rapidly in teaching her abdominal respiration, but the superb organ of the cantatrice was not long in submitting to the *contre-coup* of this transformation.

CHAPTER VI.

ABDOMINAL RESPIRATION.

It permits the storing of a volume of air greater than by clavicular respiration; but it utilises only the contraction of the diaphragm, and leaves the thoracic muscles inactive.—Whatever may be the method of respiration, muscular fatigue is in direct ratio with the effect produced ; it is manifested less quickly when the work is divided between a greater number of agents.—Why has Nature endowed us with a movable thorax if this ought to remain in a condition of fixity in the deep inspirations required by the act of singing ?—Abdominal respiration submits the stomach, the uterus, and the other viscera to strong pressure, and morbid accidents occur in consequence.

WHILE in the clavicular type the dilatation of the chest is produced principally by movements forwards and upwards of the sternum—that is to say, by increase in its antero-posterior diameter—it is, on the contrary, determined in the abdominal type by the contraction of the diaphragm and the lengthening of its vertical diameter.

But it is sufficient to consider the conical form of the thorax in order to deduce the fact, *à priori,* that the large muscular septum which serves as its base can much more augment the dimensions of the chest than can the separation of the ribs at the summit.

It is, moreover, easy to determine this point by means of the spirometer. The researches which we have made with this instrument, and which are mentioned further on, can leave no doubt upon this subject. Abdominal respiration gives to the singer the faculty of introducing into his lungs a volume of air greater than that furnished by clavicular respiration.

Our excellent friend, Mr. Lennox Browne, who has measured the thoracic cavity in the different respiratory types, arrives at a similar conclusion, which will be found set forth in the remarkable work which he has published in collaboration with M. Behnke.* The spirometric figures which he has obtained in individuals who protrude the abdomen, are much higher than among people who raise the

* *Voice, Song, and Speech.* London, 1891.

shoulders and the clavicle. That, says our distinguished *confrère*, is a fact which cannot be disputed by any kind of argument, and which is sufficient in itself to weigh the balance down upon the side of abdominal respiration. And recently* Mr. Lennox Browne cited very conclusive cases of two subjects respiring with the upper portion of the chest in whom the spirometer indicated figures below the average capacity. Their education was undertaken ; at the end of a few lessons they practised the abdominal method comfortably, and their respiratory capacity had increased more than sixty cubic inches. There is, therefore, no discussion possible on this point ; the abdominal type has the advantage over the clavicular of putting more wind (*souffle*) at the disposal of the singer ; but we shall see, on the contrary, that, compared with the costal method, it possesses a distinct inferiority in this respect.

Now, like the superior costal type, abdominal respiration presents the grave inconvenience of being only a *partial respiration*, localised at a single region of the chest, namely, at its base. But in singing, inspiratory am-

* British Laryngological and Rhinological Association, March 9th, 1892.

plification ought to take place over the whole
of the thoracic cavity.

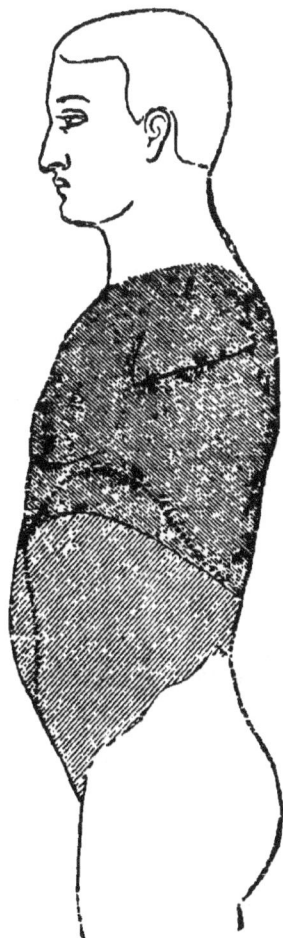

FIG. 5.
Abdominal type. The dotted line represents the condition
before inspiration.

This is a reason which should cause us to
reject the employment of the abdominal type,

5

that is to say, of every respiratory method ;
(1) which enjoins inspiration by the swelling
of the abdomen ; (2) resulting from the contraction of the diaphragm only, without the
help of the external inspiratory muscles.

The walls of the abdomen are pushed
forward by the viscera contained in the
abdominal cavity, at the expense of which
the thoracic dilatation is effected. The lower
ribs remain almost immovable ; there is no
lateral enlargement, such as we observe in the
costal method, and the viscera cannot be
lodged in the hypochondria. The abdomen
protrudes the more over the median line as
the movement of descent of the diaphragm is
the more pronounced.

The external inspiratory forces, moreover,
do not intervene ; the muscles of the thoracic
wall, which have the function of elevating the
ribs, remain at rest. The work of the diaphragm is alone brought into play. It is this
which Mandl himself endeavours to establish.*

" _One muscle only_," says he, " acts in inspiration ; it enlarges the vertical diameter of the
thorax. The force expended to put it in

* _De la fatigue de la voix_, p. 15. Paris, 1885 :
Labbé, éditeur.

movement is minimal, for it is expended only in the displacement of the soft and movable viscera of the abdominal cavity. When, for the needs of singing, a prolonged aspiration is necessary, the struggle between the inspiratory and the expiratory muscles *is exerted entirely* upon the same viscera, and the thoracic walls *experience no fatigue.*"

And again : " Abdominal respiration exacts *complete lowering* of the diaphragm.[*] We can affirm that the contraction of the diaphragm is always accompanied with the elevation of the ribs, and it has been desired to explain this displacement in various manners. But when the person is completely master of diaphragmatic respiration, deep inspirations can be taken *without elevating the ribs in any manner*, as Magendie has already said.[†]

We have reproduced these quotations in order to defend ourselves from the reproach which has been addressed to us by M. Weber[‡] —namely, that of having attributed to Mandl opinions which he did not profess.

The preceding lines make it quite intelli-

[*] *De la fatigue de la voix*, p. 15. Paris, 1855: Labbé, éditeur.

[†] *Ibid.*, p. 6.

[‡] *Le Temps*, July 20th, 1892.

gible how this author comprehends the abdominal type, without the participation of the thoracic muscles and without the elevation of the ribs ; since, according to him, *one muscle alone acts*, namely, the diaphragm, which is *completely lowered*; since the vocal struggle is strictly limited to this same diaphragm and the abdominal expiratory muscles ; and since people who are perfect masters of this respiratory method can make deep inspirations without raising the ribs.

We do not ignore the fact that Mandl has also said "that the respiratory types may be combined "; but that is another question.

We have never dreamt of denying that the diaphragm is capable of superadding its action to the external inspiratory muscles ; but then it is no longer the abdominal method, but the costal, in which we find flattening, and not protuberance, of the abdomen. The lowering of the diaphragm is moderate, and consecutive to the movement of the elevation of the ribs.

If Mandl has so much insisted upon the isolated contraction of the diaphragm, it is to give force to an important argument for the defenders of the abdominal type—to wit, that

the fatigue of the thoracic muscles is reduced
to nothing in this respiratory method.

We cannot admit this view, for we have not
observed any particular fatigue in subjects
who do not breathe with the abdomen, at
least, so long as they do not surpass the limits
of their power, in making excessive and exaggerated inspirations ; fatigue supervenes
then, by reason of the effort produced, and
this is the case with all methods of respiration.

For the rest, it is a common accusation,
which can be advanced equally well by the
adversaries of each type.   Thus, Dr. Cheval,*
after having remarked that when the thorax
is raised its return to the state of repose is
facilitated by the weight and elasticity of its
parts, writes :—

" In the abdominal method, the weight inter-
venes, on the contrary, to oppose the ascensional movement of the diaphragm ; the
stomach and the liver, which weigh two kilos,
strongly pushed down by the energetic contraction of the diaphragm, are not raised again
by the elastic retraction of the abdominal
walls, which would be much too slow, but by
an energetic muscular contraction.   The

* Bonheur, *loc. cit.*

epigastric depression ought to fly as before a blow, said Mandl."

We read again, in the same work : " We can attribute to the abdominal type excessive fatigue and 'holes' in the voice. The path which Mandl would make the nervous current flow, to cause inspiration by the contraction of the abdominal muscles, exacts a disproportionate expense of energy, by the putting into action of a long nervous chain and muscular masses not habituated to this work, and again an energetic inspiratory contraction is succeeded by an expiratory contraction if possible more energetic still."

We guard ourselves from assuming the responsibility of such opinions. If we have reproduced these lines it is with the object of impartiality.

After having shown that professors in opposition accuse each other of the same crimes, we shall put these adversaries back to back, stating that, in spite of everything, the abdominal method is capable of giving excellent results, as, for example, in the case of M. Faure.

The important point in respiratory mechanics, as in everything else, is for the singer not to go beyond his capabilities, not to abuse his strength, and to regulate his movements perfectly, in default of which he courts the risk of causing injury to the regular play of the function.

Let us, then, leave on one side this question of fatigue, and let us ask if it is logical and profitable to utilise the contraction of the diaphragm alone, when we have at our disposal the precious help of the muscles of the thoracic walls.

What should impel us to augment only the vertical diameter of the chest, and to bring only one single agent into function? The expenditure of strength necessary for the production of sound being spread over many muscles, will not the work of each of them be less?

And as the illustrious author of *l'Usage des Parties* has said, why has not Nature, so wise, so foreseeing, enclosed the heart and lungs in an osseous box, like the cranium ; why has she endowed us with a movable thoracic cage, if the envelope of the chest must always remain in the same condition of fixity? If the sternum, clavicle, ribs, and the dorsal vertebræ possess articular surfaces, it is in order that there may be movements between these osseous parts, unless these latter are all joined together, as by ankylosis. But, it being admitted that there are movements, and that the chest is dilated and contracted, how can we suppose that the thorax ought to remain immovable in an act such as singing, which necessitates great respiratory amplitudes ?

In calm inspiration, which has for its aim simply to renew the air of the pulmonary vesicles, to convey the fuel indispensable to the phenomena of combustion, the diaphragm may serve for all that is needed. But when it is a case of taking in as much air as possible, of maintaining this air at a certain pressure, of regulating and managing its exit, it is necessary to bring to its aid the inspiratory and expiratory costal forces. To maintain the contrary is to deny evidence, and to admit the complete inutility of the thoracic apparatus.

We have seen, moreover, that our most eminent physiologists have proved the participation of the thoracic walls in great respiratory movements. We have, moreover, related the experiments of Marcy, Chassagne, and Dally, showing that the chest is de-

veloped under the influence of those gym-
nastic exercises which call forth profound
inspirations.

It would appear to us, then, to be established
that in singing it is necessary to raise the ribs
by means of the external inspiratory muscles,
in default of which, as we shall see immediately,
the pectoral cavity is not enlarged in its
greatest diameter, namely, the transverse, and
can only fulfil imperfectly its office of sound
cavity.

There is also another inconvenience, quite
as serious, which results from the employment
of the abdominal type—viz., that of submitting
to a strong pressure the organs enclosed in
the abdominal cavity, and thus of provoking
different morbid accidents.

In this method of respiration the expiratory
force is furnished by the muscles of the abdominal walls, which contract energetically,
pressing upwards the intestines, the stomach,
the liver, and the spleen. But the diaphragm
is still strongly lowered, and must continue to
be maintained in a condition of contraction,
in order to prevent the too sudden exit of air.
It follows that in spite of the elasticity of the
intestinal gases, the abdominal viscera cannot

escape the combined pressure of the inspiratory and expiratory forces.

" What lost work," says Cheval, " to push in every sense the intestinal mass which tends to exit by the natural and artificial orifices; how many hernias, what affections of the liver and stomach, what troubles of the abdominal circulation, cannot such a manœuvre produce, and what digestions must this trituration lead to ? "

Far be it from us to maintain that such accidents are manifested in all who breathe with the abdomen. Clinical observation daily enforces upon us opposition to such a contention. But we are obliged to recognise that in subjects so predisposed the abdominal method may be the origin of the symptoms indicated, and in two cases doubt has not seemed possible as to the true origin of the affection.

The first case was that of a young person twenty-two years of age, perfectly normal and in good health, who had been able to sing with impunity up to the day when she fell into the hands of a fanatical professor of abdominal respiration. After two months of such instruction, dysmenorrhœic troubles appeared ; she then began to suffer persistent pain in the lower part of the abdomen, and walking became very painful. We discovered a retroversion of the uterus. Appropriate treatment, and change of professor, led to cessation of these symptoms, which have not since recurred.

The second case was that of a young woman twenty-one years of age, who had always enjoyed excellent health and had never suffered with the stomach. She began to study singing with a master who obliged her to breathe with the abdomen. It was not long before she experienced imperfect digestion, with drowsiness, flatulence, and acid risings. Then the appetite disappeared, and a sharp pain was felt at intervals in the epigastric region and between the shoulders. Then repeated vomitings occurred, hindering alimentation ; the unhappy patient could not even support milk diet, and became depressed almost to melancholy. All treatment was a failure up to the time when she abandoned not only the abdominal method, but the professor as well. After a year of rest this lady has again begun to sing, employing costal respiration, and she has had no more gastric complaints.

In 1880 Dr. Wing * also called attention to the hurtful consequences of abdominal respiration, and he related the cases of four young women previously in good health, who became invalids after some months of practice with abdominal respiration. One was affected with uterine displacement, another was attacked with leucorrhœa and lumbar pains during walking ; and dysmenorrhœic affections appeared in the two latter, although menstruation formerly had been quite painless.

In reference to this the same author quotes the words of a professor to a pupil who complained of not being able to walk since she had followed his lessons : " An artist who wishes to sing ought to expect to be no longer able to walk."

Dr. Barnes, an American gynæcologist, quoted by Wing, has also observed disorders of the same nature in women who swell out the abdomen in inspiration, and he remarked that uterine prolapse is often the result of the abdominal method of breathing.

Inguinal or crural hernias, varicoceles will also come under notice, and while admitting

* Boston *Med. and Surg. Journal*, 1880.

that these accidents only occur in isolated cases, it will be wise to attentively watch the employment of the method of abdominal respiration.

However, in spite of these multiple inconveniences, the doctrine of Mandl has been defended by men whose scientific and artistic authority is incontestable.

Among physicians we find Ch. Battaille, Ed. Fournié, Béclard, Debay, Vacher, Lermoyez, Gouguenheim, Langmaid, Nuvoli, Masucci; among writers upon musical subjects, J. Weber, Gustave Bertrand, Delprat, J. F. Bernard, Henri Lavoix; among professors, Panofka, Holtzem, Concone, Batiste, Audubert, Crosti, Lemaire, Giraudet, Mme. Marchesi, and Faure, who writes in his remarkable treatise :— *

" From the singer's point of view, we ought to endeavour to respire just as in the state of sleep when placed in a horizontal position. Abdominal respiration, which ought to be preferred to thoracic respiration, is the only method which allows the storing up of a large quantity of air without leading to any kind of contortion, such as, for example, the

* *Méthode de Chant.* Paris : Heugel, éditeur.

too frequent raising of the shoulders at each inspiration ; it permits the singer to obtain instantaneous attack in the ' demi-appel ' and in the ' quarts d'appel ' of the air blast, without disturbing the most lively movements of the theme."

We shall be only too happy if, with such numerous and eminent opponents, we succeed in causing the abandonment of the practice of abdominal breathing, and the adoption of costal respiration, which we are now going to study.

CHAPTER VII.

COSTAL RESPIRATION.

The movement of dilatation is general; the chest participates in its entirety in inspiratory amplification. The thorax is everywhere enlarged in its greatest diameter, viz., the transverse. Geometrical formula relative to the estimation of the thoracic volume. Spirometric researches establish the fact that, with the costal method, the greatest quantity of air is placed at the disposal of the singer.

WE have insisted upon the great inconvenience presented by the clavicular and abdominal methods of being only partial respiration of the summit or the base of the thorax, augmenting either the antero-posterior diameter or the vertical diameter of the chest.

In the costal method we have, on the contrary, to do with general respiration, the maximum action of which takes place over the middle region of the thorax. It is in its transverse diameter that this latter is enlarged the most ; nevertheless, all the ribs, save the two or three uppermost, are pushed upwards and outwards in inspiration, while the convexity of the diaphragm tends to be effaced.

The movement of dilatation is not localised to one part of the chest; the latter in its entirety participates in the inspiratory expansion, which being generalised will not be more exaggerated at the base than at the summit, from whence follows over these regions a diminution in the muscular expenditure which is shared between a great number of agents.

This costal respiration is, besides, that form which most augments the capacity of the thoracic reservoir; there is, therefore, no need to set forth the precious advantages which result to an artist of having at his disposal a great quantity of air, and of being able to perform musical phrases of long duration.

" A singer," said the method of the Conservatoire, "who has not exercised the art of respiration will be forced to breathe frequently, but his powers will be soon exhausted, and his voice will be heard only in feeble and vacillating sounds. Without a great volume of air, which he ought to know how to retain and manage for a long time with ability, there is no force or tone in the voice; moreover, without this faculty it is scarcely possible to phrase well in singing."

The costal type permits of the most abundant provision of air, because the transverse diameter of the chest, which is thereby increased, is the most extensive, and develops more greatly the dimensions of the lungs.

"The three diameters of the lungs," said Sappey,* "differ much in their importance ; the transverse notably exceeds the two others. This is why the lengthening of one of these diameters, or even of both, cannot suffice to compensate entirely for the lengthening of the first." It is this which leads us to maintain that the dilatation of the chest in its lateral sense constitutes the most important movement of the respiratory mechanism in respect of the air to be utilised.

Our excellent confrère, Mr. Mayo Collier, of London, one of the warmest supporters of thoracic respiration, demonstrates the point in question in a very ingenious fashion, basing his argument upon a geometrical theorem.

It suffices to recall the fact that the chest has been compared to a cone, of which the base corresponds to the diaphragm, and to

* *Traité d'anatomie.*

apply to the valuation of its volume the well-known formula :

$$V = \frac{h}{3} \pi r^2$$

V representing the capacity of the thorax ;

h the height of the cone—that is to say, the vertical diameter ;

r the radius of the base ;

π the relation between the diameter of the circle and its circumference.

A simple glance at this equation makes it intelligible that if *h* is augmented by the lowering of the diaphragm, it will, however, always be divided by 3, so that in every case the increase of *h* cannot influence in any sensible manner the volume of the cone when the surface of the base πr^2 is not modified.

On the contrary, an increase, however feeble, of *r* will always have great importance, since, in the formula, *r* is *squared*.

Supposing the lengthening of *h* may reach four centimètres, a figure in excess of reality, and that the greatest maximum of the diameter remains the same—that is to say, two centimètres for *r*.

We shall have for the abdominal type : —

$$V = \frac{h+4}{3} \pi^2$$

And for the costal type :—

$$V = \frac{h}{3} \pi (r+2)^2$$

A simple calculation will give figures mathematically establishing the following fact : the descent of the diaphragm has much less effect upon the thoracic capacity than the outward movement of the costal apparatus.

The employment of the spirometer furnishes similar results.

Certain authors, Béclard and Lennox Browne among others, have maintained that the abdominal type procures for the singer the greatest volume of air, but this was comparatively to the clavicular type, and upon this point we can only state our agreement with them. If, on the contrary, we bring the costal method into comparison, it must be admitted that the advantage remains with the latter.

Miss Pollard,* who has studied with the spirometer the volumetric relations between

* *Journal of Physiology.* Cambridge, March, 1890.

the abdominal and costal methods, draws
from her numerous experiments these conclusions : the figures obtained establish the fact

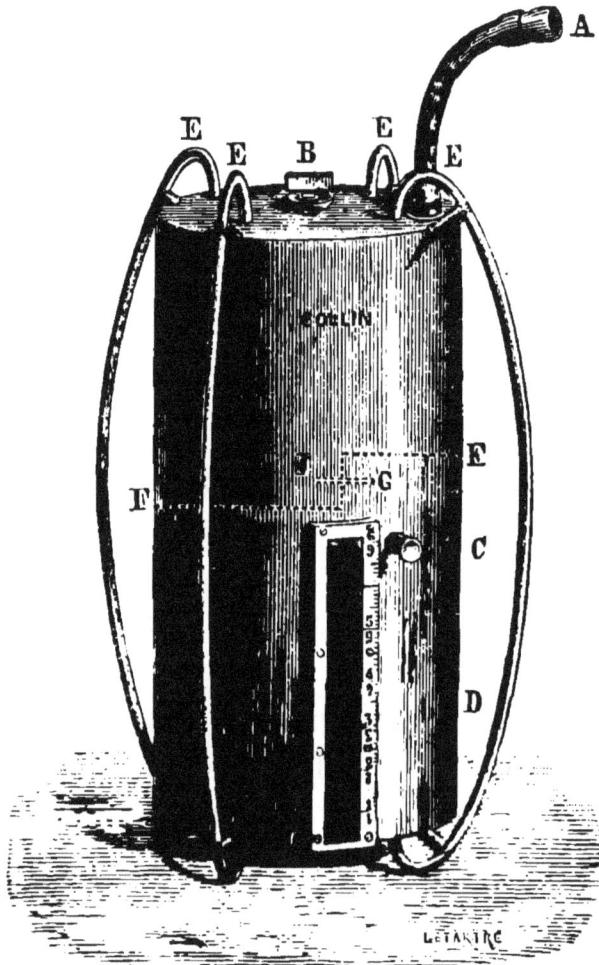

FIG. 6.—Spirometer.

that in the same individual the vital capacity
is less in abdominal respiration than in costal.

The researches which we have ourselves undertaken permit us also to be quite affirmative upon this point.

We have measured the volume of air expired, by means of the spirometer which we have devised, and of which a detailed description will be found in a former work,* and from which we reproduce the illustration. Let us content ourselves in this place with stating that this instrument has a double Mariotte's vase, composed of two chambers placed over one another and separated by two semi-circular diaphragms, F H, which are joined by a vertical septum. The two chambers are put into communication by a tube, I. The apparatus being half full of water, and the liquid filling the upper reservoir, if we breathe by the mouthpiece A, a quantity of water is displaced, and flows out of the upper reservoir into the lower one ; the graduated glass permitting us to determine the level of the liquid.

When the upper chamber is empty it suffices to turn the instrument upside down, corking the tube E, and placing the mouthpiece A on the chamber D, at the same time

* *Revue de Laryngologie et d'Otologie.* Bordeaux, April, May, 1890.

that we raise the screw C, and close the opening C. The instrument once started can continue its action indefinitely, offering the important advantage of opposing to the expired air a resistance equal to all the momenta of the experiment.

In our experiments all the subjects have at first, for a few initial sittings, merely learned how to use our instrument. That is a practical point which it is necessary not to forget, for there is generally only need of a little ability and a few trials to see the first figure of the indicated scale mount, without the vital capacity having really been augmented.

The numbers which we record represent the average results furnished by each individual, and on each we have repeated our experiments fifteen times.

The first series of researches had for its aim the measurement of the volume of air expired by the same person according as that person used the clavicular or costal type of respiration. For this we chose adult women of from twenty to thirty years of age, belonging to all conditions, but who had never studied singing, and in whom the clavicular mode of breathing was very characteristic,

After making large inspirations, the spirometer gave us the quantities of air rejected
by forced expiration.

Then we caused the respiratory type to
change; we made these individuals immobilise
the summit of the thorax, and depress the
abdomen so as to enlarge the middle and
inferior parts of the chest. In this education
we have never met with any serious difficulty.
After some days or weeks, when the costal
respiration was correctly practised, we took
fresh spirometrical measurements.

We experimented in this way on twenty-
three women, and proved that the costal
method determined an increase of —

700 to 800	cubic centimètres of air in			2
600 to 700	,,	,,	,,	5
500 to 600	,,	,,	,,	6
400 to 500	,,	,,	,,	4
300 to 400	,,	,,	,,	2
200 to 300	,,	,,	,,	1
100 to 200	,,	,,	,,	3

In a second series of experiments we grouped
twelve subjects of the feminine sex, who had
undergone vocal studies, and whose respiration
had been already transformed by professors.
These persons had arrived at the point of no

longer making use of the costal type in singing, but it was, nevertheless, easy for them to
employ on occasion the clavicular method.
We have been enabled by means of the spirometer to compare the proportions of air
utilised by each system.   We have noted
that the costal type produced an augmentation of—

600 to 700 cubic centimètres in 3 subjects.
500 to 600   „   „   4   „
400 to 500   „   „   1 subject.
300 to 400   „   „   3 subjects.
200 to 300   „   „   1 subject.

We are, then, justified in maintaining that
the vital capacity is greater with the costal
type of breathing than with the clavicular
type.

Fifteen adult individuals of the masculine
sex, not taken from singers, served for our
third series of experiments.   It was desired
to know the volumetric variations occasioned
by the abdominal and costal methods.   In the
ordinary condition these subjects respired by
swelling the abdomen.   Their spirometric
measurement was taken, the ribs remaining
immovable.   They then succeeded pretty
rapidly in thoroughly dilating the base of the

thorax, making use of a belt to slightly compress the abdomen. The quantity of air was increased in costal respiration, from—

300 to 400 cubic centimètres in 5 individuals.
200 to 300 „   „   6   „
100 to 200 „   „   2   „

In two cases we noted negative results, without having been able to determine the cause which could explain these exceptions.

A fourth series comprised seven men, lyric artists, breathing by the costal method during singing, and advancing, on the contrary, the abdomen in normal inspirations. We found in favour of the costal method a difference of—

600 to 700 cubic centimètres in 2 individuals.
500 to 600 „   „   3   „
400 to 500 „   „   1 individual.
300 to 400 „   „   1   „

Lastly, in three singers, perfect masters of their respiratory movements, and able to employ at will either one of the three types, but more familiar with the costal method, which they used ordinarily in singing, we registered the following average measurements :—

Clavicular Resp.	Abdominal Resp.	Costal Resp.
4,600 cubic cent.	5,200 cubic cent.	5,300 cubic cent.
4,000 „ „	4,300 „ „	4,800 „ „
3,700 „ „	4,000 „ „	4,300 „ „

The figures indicated prove beyond a doubt the fact that we desire to establish—viz., that costal respiration puts at the disposal of the singer a greater quantity of air than the clavicular and abdominal methods.

CHAPTER VIII.

COSTAL RESPIRATION—Continued.

The artist can regulate with precision the exit of the
air-blast.—Vocal effort, muscular antagonism, and
synergy.—Insufficiency of the abdominal powers.—
Respiratory mechanism of the *"son filé."* *—Thoracic
resonance : the sounding properties of the pectoral
cavity are brought out by the costal type.

I T does not suffice merely to accumulate a
large quantity of air ; it is equally in-
dispensible for the singer to know thoroughly
how to economise his air-blast (*souffle*) and to
utilise it only in proportion to his vocal needs.
The artist ought to endeavour to make himself
completely master of his respiration, and ought
to learn how to retain his breath as much as
possible, and to retard as much as possible the
retraction and falling back of the expanded
chest.

* To *filer un son—i.e.,* to draw out a tone—is equivalent to the Italian *" mezza di voce,"* literally, half the
power of the voice.—TRANSLATOR.

" In singing," says Paul Bert,[*] "expiration slowly, and, by professional singers, wisely regulated and controlled, allows only the escape of such a quantity of air as is in relation with the energy of the laryngeal vibrations. To allow the escape through the glottis of only such a volume of air as is precisely necessary to produce the desired effect, is one of the difficulties of the singer's art."

It can be conceived that if respiration is short, if the provision of air, although abundant, is rapidly dissipated, it becomes impossible to maintain or graduate a sound, to add grace or artistic effect to the singing. The most beautiful voices are then deprived of charm, and produce no impression upon the hearer.

" In the old Italian school," say MM. Lemaire and Lavoix,[†] "the singer looked for his effect especially in the extent and flexibility of the voice, always sure of exciting more pleasure and enthusiasm by a beautiful *mezza di voce*, by trills, and by all the brilliant embellishments with which he enriched his singing, rather than by violent efforts of passion. It was chiefly to the art of breathing well that

[*] *Leçons sur la Respiration.* Paris, 1870.
[†] *Loc. cit.*

he owed the sweetness, the purity, and the endurance of his voice ; he also learned with the greatest care to economise his respiration, to the extent of being able to execute passages the duration of which exceeded seventy to seventy-five seconds. Farinelli, for example, sang passages composed of three hundred notes without taking breath."

It is therefore necessary in the highest degree to accurately gauge the expiratory movement, in order to regulate with precision the exit of the air. By the costal type this can be more easily accomplished than by the abdominal method, in which the thoracic muscles are allowed to be inactive.

It is well known that the mechanical phenomena of respiration are dependent upon two orders of muscles, and that in the act of singing there is a struggle, and an opposition, between the inspiratory and expiratory agents. The chest is first dilated by the inspiratory muscles. These latter, instead of ceasing to act, continue to contract more or less energetically, so as to retain the air in the lungs, which otherwise would be rapidly driven out by the expiratory muscles.

Mandl maintains that the struggle is chiefly

in the abdominal cavity, where meet the antagonistic forces of the diaphragm and the muscles of the abdominal wall. We believe, on the contrary, that the struggle occurs principally between the muscles which unite the different portions of the thorax, the abdominal muscles playing a secondary part ; and we base our opinion upon the physiological ideas of the *effort* which is evident in all expiratory movements of a certain duration, and which can only be caused by the action of the thoracic muscles.

Professor Ledentu says, in his remarkable article in the *Dictionary of Medicine and Surgery* : *

"The true characteristic of effort is that, whatever may be the modification to which respiration submits, we can always demonstrate that the thorax is immobilised completely or incompletely, either totally or partially, in different cases. Thus the effort offers certain varieties. There are efforts which are almost entirely limited to the thorax, such as of crying, *singing*, coughing ; they are executed only according to a particular modification impressed upon the flow of air outwards from

* *Effort*, t. xii.

the lungs. These are expirations of a special type, accompanied with an unaccustomed display of strength, and with vocal phenomena of diverse natures."

Adopting the ideas of Verneuil,* this author admits three kinds of efforts :—

1. *General*, or *thoracic*, or *abdominal* effort, in which there is closure of the four sphincters, which allow the passage of alimentary and fæcal matters, urine, and air ; this is effort properly so called.

2. *Abdominal*, or *expulsive* effort, in which the expiratory muscles play the principal part, retracting the abdominal or thoracic cavity in all diameters. Here some of the sphincters are closed, while the others are opened, to permit the passage of air, urine, fæces, etc.

3. *Thoracic* effort, in which respiration is not suspended, and which consists not only in energetic and sudden contraction of the external dilating muscles of the thorax, but in the continuation and persistence of this contraction.

It is to this variety that vocal effort belongs. The qualifications, *abdominal* and *thoracic*, which Verneuil employed to designate the

* *Société de Chirurgie.* Paris, 1856.

two latter kinds of effort, clearly show that in the expulsive efforts of crying, micturition, and vomiting, the abdominal muscles intervene incessantly, while in vocal effort the action of the thoracic muscles predominates, which means that, in singing, as we maintain, abdominal effort ought to hold a secondary place, and that the bulk of the action ought to be especially supported by the thoracic powers chiefly.

" At the commencement of their studies," said Ledentu, " singers do not know yet how to maintain the contraction of the external inspiratory muscles while they relax the diaphragm in order to emit sound. They have short breath, and *lose all their wind* in a few moments. Later on, when exercises have taught them that the best manner of retarding expiration is to maintain as long as possible the fixity of the thorax, they realise, without knowing it, thoracic effort."

If, indeed, the inspiratory muscles and the external expiratory muscles are contracted with equal intensity, the thorax is fixed, and expiration can be performed by the relaxation of the diaphragm alone ; but then the column of air is expelled too feebly to produce sonorous vibrations of the vocal cords. In this case only a very feeble and very gentle sound would be produced : this is what occurs when a person hums.

If it is wished to emit a stronger sound it is necessary to accentuate the contraction of the thoracic expirators, so that their action may surpass that of their antagonistic muscles, the inspirators. When the note has to be emitted with as much intensity as possible, the expirators will be contracted to their maximum degree, and the inspirators to their minimum.

This mechanism of vocal effort is very well explained by Hamonic,* who concludes by saying : " The singer must exercise himself in contracting singly the inspiratory and expiratory muscles, and in making them act with equal or unequal force, so as to obtain with them that kind of functional independence which is the secret of vocal effort."

Let us now suppose an artist who wishes to graduate a sound, that is to say, to produce the vocal effect called *mezza di voce* by Italians, attacking the note at first *pianissimo*, and gradually passing through all the shades of

* *Manuel du Chanteur* Paris, 1888.

7

crescendo, to end in *forte*, and return through *diminuendo* to *pianissimo* again. This singer having filled his chest with air according to the costal method, will continue to contract his inspiratory muscles in such a manner that the action of the expiratory muscles may in some degree be neutralised, and so that the sound emitted may be very feeble. The energy of these latter then increases progressively, while that of the inspiratory muscles diminishes, which will be at its minimum at the moment of *forte*, the precise moment when, on the contrary, the power of the expiratory muscles would be at its maximum. In the period of decrease of the *mezza di voce* the same phenomena are produced in the inverse order ; at the final *pianissimo* the action of the inspiratory muscles would become almost equal to that of the expiratory muscles.

In Mandl's system, the abdominal muscles contracting during expiration, the resistance will be represented by the diaphragm ; but according to physiological laws of *synergy* and muscular *antagonism*, every movement, to be perfectly regulated, demands the putting into play of the entire group destined to accomplish it ; so much so, that in the inspiratory group, the thoracic dilators remaining inactive, it may be asked whether with the contraction alone of the diaphragm, the expulsion of air is regulated with such precision as by the costal method.

There can be no doubt as to the answer, and observers have signalised this serious inconvenience of the abdominal type, without, however, assigning the reason.

"In breathing with flat or concave abdomen," says Morell Mackenzie,* there is far more control over expiration than when the diaphragm is displaced ; the act can be regulated absolutely by the will to suit the requirements of the vocalist. Abdominal inspiration is apt, on the other hand, to be followed by jerky expiration, a defect which is fatal to artistic delivery and most fatiguing to the singer."

These lines are added to a note written by Mr. Mayo Collier, who thus expresses his opinion : "Gottfried Weber,† one of the most acute investigators who has studied the

* *Hygiene of the Vocal Organs*, Seventh Edition, p. 96. 1890.
† *Cæcilia*, 1835, t. xvii.

science of singing, says that undoubtedly the old Italian method is the best.

"We agree with Gottfried Weber that the method of the old school is the best, and that by it more air can be taken in, more complete control maintained over the expiratory act, and waste more efficiently prevented. . . . In the convex form (abdominal inspiration) there is no means of regulating the relaxation of the diaphragm, and so economising the air in the lungs."

Cheval * also speaks of the intermittent and irregular exit of the air in the system taught by Mandl.

With costal respiration the singer can then dispose of a greater quantity of air, and can measure its outflow exactly ; he can, besides, bring out the full resonant properties of the chest, considered as a sounding-box.

It is of greater importance to insist upon this last point, inasmuch as it has been overlooked by most authors.

The qualities of the voice, principally the intensity and the tone, depend not only upon the vibrations of the inferior vocal cords, but also upon the vibrations of the air in

* Bonheur *loc. cit.*

the sonorous chambers situated above and below the larynx. Since the beautiful discoveries of Helmholtz upon the harmonics of the fundamental sound, and upon the formation of the vowels, it has been generally accepted that the ventricles of the larynx, the pharynx, the mouth, the nasal fossæ, and the accessory sinuses, act as resonators, and determine the tone of the voice. On the contrary, with the exception of Edouard Fournié, de Koch, Nitot, Gouguenheim, Lermoyez, Sewal, and Pollard, physiologists do not seem to have given attention to the thorax as a sounding-box.

However, the old expressions of *head voice* and *chest voice* indicate well that for a long time certain characters of the chest register have been attributed to the vocal modifications imparted by the vibrations of the thorax and its contents.

"When a violin resounds," say Gouguenheim and Lermoyez,* "no one can deny that the sound is produced by the vibration of the cord which the bow strikes ; why, then, is it that when this cord vibrates the air over such a small area the sound which results has sometimes

* *Physiologie de la voix et de chant.* Paris, 1885.

an extreme intensity? Because below the cord there is a sounding-box which vibrates in unison with this cord, and which agitates the air over a large surface. Similarly below the vocal cords, which we concede produce a weak and feeble sound, there is an enormous resonant cavity constituted by the thorax, the lungs, and the trachea, and which gives to the voice all the intensity which it needs."

In order to demonstrate the vibrations of the thoracic walls, it is sufficient to place the palm of the hand over the chest of an individual who is speaking ; there is then felt a sensation which can leave no doubt in any mind, and the variations which these symptoms submit to in certain morbid conditions furnish the physician with a valuable element of diagnosis.

These vibrations are not perceived with the same clearness throughout the whole extent of the thorax ; there is ordinarily a maximum centre which changes its localisation, according as the sound is low or acute. In general, according as the tone rises, this vibratory nucleus rises from the base to the middle part of the thorax, and from this to the summit. When the chest voice is transformed into the head voice, the vibrations of the base disappear almost completely, and the vocal *fremitus* becomes perceptible only in the supra-spinous and sub-clavicular fossæ. Then, for example, while the note la^2 * provokes vibrations of the whole depth of the chest, the si^2 will find its maximum nucleus at the level of the sternum, the ut^3 little higher, and so on up to la^3 ; at the moment of emission of this note it is the supra-laryngeal portions of the vocal tube which are put into vibration.

"The larynx," says Edouard Fournié,† "possesses an especial table of harmonics ; but, in this respect, it is distinguished from other instruments by the remarkable particularity, that the resounding cavity can change its form and dimensions according to the note emitted. Here is a marvellous phenomenon, and one which art has never been able to imitate ! To each note corresponds a particular table of harmonics which re-enforce the sound with so much the more exactitude

---

* The French musical notation is—do (*or* ut), ré, mi, fa, sol, la, si ; and the corresponding English notation, is : c, d, e, f, g, a, b ; the numbers over the notes, *e.g.*, la^2, ut^3, etc., indicate the octaves.

† *Physiologie de la Voix.* Paris, 1866.

and clearness, as this adaptation is not under the dependence of the will of the singer. In man the harmonic table is situated over the whole course of the aërial passages, from the pulmonary vesiculi up to the lips, and without the singer occupying himself with it, each note finds in this long passage the resounding part which is most appropriate for its re-enforcement."

Fournié, therefore, considers the thorax to be a veritable resounding cavity ; and it has been a matter of regret to us not to find any trace of the doctrines of this French physician in the recent study which Sewal and Pollard † have published on this question.

The American scientists have undertaken a series of researches, with the aim of establishing the fact that during phonation the thorax behaves as a resonator, and that the form and the capacity of the pectoral cavity contribute to impress upon the voice its qualities, and to raise or lower the sounds emitted by the vocal cords.

They have observed that in mounting the scale, acute notes are emitted more easily, with greater purity and brilliancy if, during

† *Journal of Physiology.* Cambridge, March, 1890.

expiration, the diaphragm rises at the same time that the superior portion of the chest dilates. On the contrary, in descending the musical scale, a lower note is obtained if, when expiration is performed by the contraction of the thorax, the diaphragm at the same time effaces its convexity. This means that a diminution in the vertical diameter of the chest, and an increase in its transverse diameter, have the effect of heightening the fundamental note of the thoracic resonator, and the diminution of the transverse diameter, and the increase of the vertical diameter lower this same note.

These experimenters demonstrate the preceding facts by the following experiment :— a bâton four feet long is held horizontally by simple pressure between the chest of an individual and an open door. To the extremity of this bâton, near to the subject, is bound a double metallic wire which descends vertically, and through the loop of which is passed another metallic thread, which is held by fixing one end to the door, and attaching a weight to the other end. The apparatus being thus applied, if the horizontal thread is made to vibrate, it is observed that the note produced differs according as the individual employs either of the expiratory processes which we have just indicated. The sound appears to be more elevated when the subject expires by relaxing his diaphragm and dilating his thorax.

Results more conclusive of the ideas of Sewal and Pollard have been obtained by means of the graphic method. Three pneumographs were applied to the same person; one above the umbilicus, the two others respectively on the sternum at the level of the eighth and fourth ribs. Tracings were taken in eighteen singers while they performed ascending and descending scales, and in four of them the tracings were very significant, and left no doubt as to the alternation of the movement of the diaphragm and ribs. It is easily recognised that in acute notes the horizontal diameter of the chest is enlarged, while the vertical diameter is diminished; and that the contrary occurs in deep sounds.

It seems, therefore, that the volume and the form of the thorax vary according to the height of sounds, and that the chest deserves to be considered as the most perfect of resonators. But in order that this latter may execute such an important function, it is, as we have seen, necessary that the thorax may have the faculty of dilating or retracting in its middle and superior portion, at the level of the eighth and fourth ribs, conditions which cannot be fulfilled if the singer employs the abdominal type, with the isolated contraction of the diaphragm, and complete inactivity of the thoracic muscles.

But let us put on one side the views of Fournié, and of Sewal and Pollard, which we have not been able experimentally to control ; let us not look upon the chest in relation to its resonance and the modifications that it has been able to imprint upon the height and tone of sounds ; let us content ourselves with Gouguenheim and Lermoyez, in considering the thorax as a simple re-enforcer of sounds, an opinion which cannot be seriously disputed. It remains not the less true that with the abdominal type this re-enforcing power cannot be fully exercised.

Indeed, the pectoral cavity being assimilated to a sounding-box, the degree of vibration of its parts will have a direct influence upon the amplitude of the undulatory movements of the air contained in the cavity, and secondly,

by the power of re-enforcement of this. No
one can ignore the fact that musical instrument makers attach the greatest value to the
nature of the wood employed in the construc-
tion of the instrument.

But the thoracic walls are built upon a
muscular and osseous plan ; the sternum, the
ribs, and some muscles which we have already
enumerated, the internal and external intercostals among others. This muscular tissue
must vibrate according to physical laws which
regulate the vibrations of cords and membranes
in general ; in a state of repose the softness
and relaxation would be unfavourable to the
production of vibrations, the formation of
these being, on the contrary, facilitated by
the contraction and tension of the muscular
fibres. It is therefore necessary, in order that
the chest may fulfil its office of re-enforcer,
that the thoracic muscles, and especially the
intercostals, which unite the ribs, should be
tense and contracted, in order to increase the
intensity of the sounds emitted in accentuating
the vibratile properties of the pectoral cavity.
This result cannot be obtained by abdominal
respiration, which utilises only the action of
the diaphragm and the walls of the abdomen.

It is quite otherwise with the costal type, which necessitates the intervention of muscular agents entering into the constitution of the walls of the thorax. The singer who employs this method, and who, in order to retain his air, moderates the action of the expiratory muscles by that of the inspiratory muscles, puts these same muscles into a state of contraction during the greatest part of the expiratory effort, and thus places the thorax in the conditions exacted by its functions as a re-enforcer of sound.

CHAPTER IX[1]

COSTAL RESPIRATION (concluded).

Movements of the ribs in costal respiration.—Function
of the diaphragm. — Doctrines of Magendie,
Duchenne, Paul Bert.—The retraction of the abdominal wall, limited to its inferior portion, favours
the elevation of the ribs by the diaphragm.—The
old Italian masters taught the costal type.—Professors and physicians who recommend this
respiratory method, and artists who practise it.

THE singer derives therefore the greatest
advantage from employing costal
respiration, and practising it according to the
following rules :—

During inspiration—

The clavicle (collar-bone) and the first rib
ought to remain immovable.

The thorax will be enlarged, especially
in its middle portion and at its base, the
point of the sternum being carried upwards
and forwards.

The depression over the stomach will follow

o

the movement of amplification of the lower ribs.

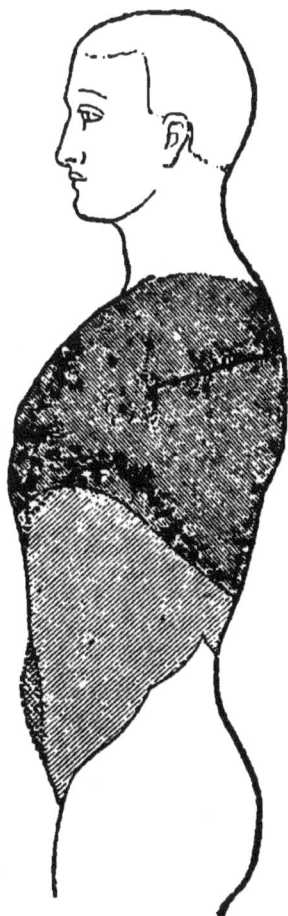

FIG. 7.
Costal type. The dotted line represents the condition before inspiration.

The abdominal wall will be slightly depressed in its inferior portion over the umbilical and hypogastric regions.

At the commencement of inspiration the scalene muscles are feebly contracted, and thus fix the first rib, which affords to the external intercostals the point of assistance necessary to enable each of these muscles to raise the rib situated below it. The thorax is at the same time elevated by the other inspiratory muscles attached to the vertebral column—that is to say, by the levatores costarum, the serratus posticus superior, and the cervicalis ascendens muscles. To the action of these muscles is added, in the most ample respirations, that of the serratus magnus, the pectoralis major, the pectoralis minor, and the latissimus dorsi (mentioned before, p. 8).

Besides, the inferior portion of the chest is equally enlarged by the diaphragm, which, in contracting, pushes the lower ribs upwards and outwards. The movement of descent of this muscle is but little pronounced, because the phrenic centre meets the abdominal viscera, which are crowded upwards by the contraction of the muscles of the abdominal walls in their two inferior thirds. These viscera offer a point of resistance to the diaphragm ; its aponeurotic portion is fixed, while its periphery, the costal insertions of which are movable, is carried upwards, which leads to the elevation of the ribs, and the increase of the antero-posterior and transverse diameters of the thorax.

Certain authors, Béclard among others, do not admit this view; they accord to the diaphragm only the power of lengthening the vertical diameter; but we do not hesitate to endorse the opinion of Beau and Maissiat, Duchenne of Boulogne, Longet, and Paul Bert, who, by their beautiful experimental researches, have been able to furnish a solid basis for the doctrine of Galien and Magendie.

The latter wrote, in his *Précis de Physiologie*:* " When the diaphragm is contracted it pushes the viscera below it ; but for that the sternum and the lower ribs would present a sufficient resistance to the effort which it makes to draw them upwards. But this resistance can only be imperfect, since all these parts are mobile. This is the reason why, each time that the diaphragm is contracted, it must always elevate the thorax more or less."

It is, moreover, demonstrated that the move-

* Duchenne de Boulogne, *Physiologie du Mouvement.* Paris, 1867.

ment of the ribs is more marked when the viscera oppose a certain resistance to the descent of the diaphragm. To be convinced of this, it suffices to have recourse to the superb pages of Duchenne of Boulogne (*Physiologie du Mouvement*).

From numerous experiments performed by this scientist the following results :—When the diaphragm is no longer in contiguity with the abdominal viscera, at the instant when it is contracted, the ribs to which it is inserted are drawn inwards, instead of being carried outwards, and the more the diaphragm is maintained in elevation during its contraction the more has it a tendency to raise the ribs.

Duchenne, exciting the phrenic nerve, has also observed that the abdominal walls offer more resistance during life than after death, and the expansion of the base of the thorax is greatest in the living animal.

And he adds : "Separation of the lower ribs by the contraction of the diaphragm increases in direct ratio to the resistance of the viscera or of the abdominal walls. This resistance, when opposed to the lowering of the diaphragm, impedes or prevents the increase of the vertical diameter of the chest ; but the transverse expansion which the chest gains then is a sort of compensation."

Paul Bert,* who has also practised numerous vivisections in order to elucidate the question, concludes in the same manner : "How is it that the fibres of the diaphragm in diminishing their convexity can raise the lower ribs? We answer, with Magendie and Duchenne, that they obtain a fulcrum from the viscera, the projection forwards of which is impeded by the abdominal walls.   If on an animal under experiment we open the abdomen, the contraction of the diaphragm no longer raises the ribs."

We are therefore in accord with the most authoritative teachings of experimental physiology in recommending to singers during inspiration to retract the abdomen, which has the effect of maintaining the viscera, and thus of furnishing a fulcrum to the diaphragm, and favouring the transverse dilatation of the thorax.

But, in the respiratory type which we teach, the flattening of the abdomen ought not to be general, or so accentuated as in the clavicular

* *Leçons sur la respiration.*

method of breathing.*   That is an important point upon which our friend John de Reszké rightly insists, advising the retraction of the abdomen only in its inferior part up to the waist, and allowing the depression over the stomach to follow the movement of costal amplification.

Let us divide as anatomists do the anterior abdominal wall into three regions :—(1) The superior or *epigastric* portion, comprised between the point of the sternum and a horizontal line joining the two lowest points of the thoracic cavity ; (2) The middle, or *umbilical*, portion, extending between the sub-costal line, and a line passing above the bones of the pelvis ; (3) The third, a lower, or *hypogastric*, region, placed between this latter limit and the pubes.

* The author and translator of this book have recently been most thoroughly misrepresented as teaching complete retraction of the abdominal walls, *i.e.*, singing with an abdomen flattened as completely as possible. Mr. Lennox Browne has credited us both with notions which we do not hold, and can scarcely have read the French edition of Dr. Joal's work, or he would surely never have been led into such a mis-statement.   The foregoing observations are a sufficient refutation of such a travesty of Dr. Joal's opinions, which, I may add, I fully endorse.—TRANSLATOR.

The umbilicus is situated about four centimètres (one and a half inches) below the subcostal line.

And let us say that it is the hypogastric and umbilical portions of the abdominal wall which ought to be elevated and slightly flattened, and that, on the contrary, the epigastric region ought to follow the movements outwards of the sternum and the costal cartilages. The compressibility of the intestinal gas intervening, the diminution of volume of the lower part of the abdomen will be easily compensated for by the increase in size of the epigastrium and of the hypochondria.

In the clavicular type of breathing the ascensional movement of the ribs is more pronounced ; the level of the diaphragmatic septum is raised ; the organs placed below this muscle, and especially the stomach, are drawn upwards, and are in *a fashion aspirated*, from whence results a very marked depression of the epigastric region, which is not observed in the costal type, where the retraction is especially sub-umbilical, and results from the contraction of the abdominal muscles, limited to their inferior fasciculi.

To resume, as to the modifications of the

abdominal walls according to the respiratory types, let us note that : (1) The clavicular method is characterised by a depression of the epigastric crease ; (2) The abdominal method by the swelling of the abdomen ; (3) The costal method by a slight flattening of the whole of the anterior abdominal region situated below the sub-costal line.*

It is now the place to remark that the term abdominal respiration is not synonymous with diaphragmatic respiration, since, in the costal type, the diaphragm also plays an important part in the increase in volume of the chest. In the same way, depression of the abdominal wall during inspiration does not involve the raising of the upper ribs, and we must protest energetically against the tendency which certain authors exhibit to range among the partisans of the clavicular type those teachers who advise the retraction of the abdomen.

We also, until the contrary is proved, believe ourselves justified in maintaining that the famous Bernacchi (of Bologna), of whom Mannstein has transmitted the teachings, that Mengozzi, and the professors who helped to establish the old method of the Conservatoire,

* For illustration see Frontispiece or Fig. 1.

employed and recommended costal respiration.

On referring to the rules contained in these
two works (*see* p. 40) it will be seen that
Bernacchi says only : " For respiration during
singing the abdomen should be retracted " ;
and that Mengozzi merely advises " flattening
the abdomen and making it re-mount with
promptitude, while swelling and advancing
the chest." These doctrines are perfectly
applicable to the costal method, so much the
more in that these illustrious singers did not
in any fashion speak of raising the shoulders.

Moreover, the celebrated Garcia seems to
us to be wrongly considered a supporter of
clavicular respiration. M. Saint-Yves Bax,
professor of the Conservatoire, an excellent
master who teaches costal respiration, has
stated to us that the great artist, of whom
he was a pupil, was on the contrary a convinced adversary of the superior costal method.
The following lines, printed in one of his
treatises,* leave no doubt upon this point, the
important *rôle* that Garcia reserves to the
diaphragm being reserved :—

" In order that air may penetrate into the

* *Méthode de chant.* Paris, 1840.

lungs," writes he, "it is necessary that the ribs should be separated and the diaphragm lowered. If in this condition the ribs are allowed to fall back and the diaphragm to be raised, the lungs, pressed on every side like a sponge in the hand, instantly abandon the air they have inspired. It is, then, necessary not to allow the ribs to fall back, and to relax the diaphragm only so much as is necessary to enforce the sound."

Our regretted teacher and friend, Sir Morell Mackenzie, who was so well versed in all vocal matters, condemns the clavicular type, " which is seldom employed except in certain diseased conditions and during very violent exertion," which, however, does not prevent this observant specialist from pronouncing clearly against the abdominal method.

"The old Italian masters taught that in inspiration the anterior abdominal wall should be slightly drawn in, and this method was practised for more than a hundred and fifty years. Signor Garcia, the lineal descendant of the old Italian school, says in his *Singing School* (chapter iv., ' On Respiration '): ' In order to inspire freely, hold the head straight, the shoulders thrown back without stiffness, and the chest open. Raise the chest by a slow and regular movement, and *draw in the stomach.'* (The *italics* are not in the original.) But in 1855 Mandl opposed this mode of breathing on anatomical grounds, maintaining that the descent of the diaphragm is facilitated by allowing the abdominal wall to be flaccid and to project forward in inspiration. Although, however, the abdominal mode of breathing may be the *natural* method of inspiration, there can, I think, be no doubt that in singing it is not the most effective."

The respiratory method taught by Morell Mackenzie is therefore the costal method, and in the last edition of his book * a note relative to this respiratory type has been added. The author of this interesting note, Mr. Mayo Collier, maintains that, during inspiration, the abdomen ought to take the concave form. We believe, however, that our distinguished *confrère* goes too far in making the statement that the abdominal walls push the diaphragm upwards; in our opinion the viscera alone serve as the fulcrum for the diaphragmatic muscles.

* *Hygiene of the Vocal Organs*, Seventh edition. 1890,

More recently Dr. Norris Wolfenden * has declared himself a supporter of the costal method, which he has expounded and defended with much talent.

Lastly, we are happy to state that we are in perfect community of opinion with Mr. Lennox Browne. The eminent former president of the British Laryngological Society desires us to make known that in the French translation of his work † he will formulate his opinion upon the matter as follows : " It is recognised that inspiration is correct when there is an increase of volume of the inferior part of the chest and upper part of the abdomen. The swelling of the abdomen ought to be limited to the epigastric region, and it ought not to extend to the hypogastrium." ‡

* *Journal of Larnygology*, June 1892.

† *Voix, Chant, et Langage.* Paris : Labonne (in the press).

‡ It is not easy always to follow Mr. Lennox Browne. Believed formerly to be an enthusiastic supporter of the abdominal method, the quotation above given would infer that he was in accord with the writer of this book. Yet he has lately published in *The Medical Week* a paper which accuses the writer and translator of advising singing with the flattened abdomen, while himself teaching

Since 1885 we have studied, outside the theatre, the respiration of eighty-five persons assiduously engaged in singing exercises, of whom sixty-two were men and twenty-three women.

Among these latter let us cite : Mesdames Albani, d'Adler, Rose Caron, Dereims, Fidès-Devriès, Dufrane, Figuet, Fursch-Madi, Leslino, Rebel, Joséphine de Reszké, and Richard. And among the men : MM. d'Andrade Frédéric Boyer, Capoul, Dereims, Dubulle Fournets, Gayarré, Gailhard, Ibos, Lassalle, Lauwers, Marris, Melchissédec, Merrit, Portejoie, Renaldi, Renaud, Jean de Reszké, Édouard de Reszké, Saléza, Sellier, Stéphanne, Talazac, Tournié, and Villaret. The other subjects

the " Protruded Abdomen," *i.e.*, the Abdominal Method. His arguments and the tone of his article would infer that he is in active opposition to the teachings of this book. We should be sorry to do any injustice to Mr. Lennox Browne, and we suppose that it must be due to our limited intelligence that we have never yet been able to comprehend his real views as to the art of breathing in singing. We admit that he speaks of expansion of the lower ribs, while teaching full descent of the diaphragm and protrusion of the abdomen, a combination of circumstances which is physiologically impossible, as the argument of the foregoing pages clearly shows.—TRANSLATOR.

were artists less eminent, or very distinguished amateurs, but all accomplished singers.

Of 23 women { 9 employed the clavicular type.
{ 14   ,,   ,,   costal type.

Of 62 men { 11   ,,   ,,   clavicular type.
{ 19   ,,   ,,   abdominal type.
{ 32   ,,   ,,   costal type.

It must be well understood that no pre-conceived idea has guided us in the choice of these subjects, with whom the accidents alone of the *clientèle*, and of ordinary circumstances, have put us into relation.

It is interesting to note that we have not met a single *chanteuse* breathing with the abdomen, although, among the twenty-three persons included in our statistics, there is one illustrious cantatrice who, according to a biography in Grove's Dictionary, had written a letter to her master, Lamperti, to felicitate the latter on the happy results furnished by the abdominal method. But we are assured that this great artist practised the costal method in all its purity.

Among men, the type which we teach is again the most frequently employed ; it was presented to our observation in thirty-two out of sixty-two cases.

We have said at the commencement of this work, that M. Jean de Reszké was a resolute defender of costal respiration. This illustrious artist, who is as learned a theoretician as he is an able practitioner, has experimented upon himself with the different respiratory methods, and has arrived at the firm conviction that the costal method, with slight depression of the abdomen in inspiration, and with entire immobility of the clavicle, is superior to all others. The singer who makes use of it commands a greater volume of air; he can retain his wind for longer, or produce more powerful vocal effects, and, lastly, he can resist fatigue much better.

M. Édouard de Reszké might serve as a model for a description of this kind. Never have we seen a chest so superb assume such a considerable volume.

M. Lasalle also declares himself clearly in favour of costal respiration, and entirely shares the views of his friend Jean de Reszké.

One of our illustrations of the French school, M. Villaret, whose long career has shone with such a brilliant light, has always breathed by raising the thorax and depressing the abdomen, without the slightest clavicular movement.   He does not doubt that this manner of breathing, "relying upon the inferior portion of the chest," aids the development and conservation of the voice.

MM. Dereims and Ibos, of the Opera, are also of this opinion ; so is M. Talzac, the worthy successor of Roger at the Opèra Comique.

Gayarré pronounced himself energetically against " the swelling of the abdomen and the raising of the shoulders."

M. Saléza has authorised us to say that at the commencement of his vocal studies he employed the abdominal type, but experience quickly revealed to him the great advantages of the costal type of respiration, which had increased the power and solidity of his voice.

Our excellent friend, the tenor Coppel, whom we have so often applauded at the Opéra Comique, and who is one of our most distinguished *confrères*, agrees that, in singing, it is necessary to respire specially with the inferior portion of the thorax.   It would be useless to contend as to the importance of all this evidence, artistic and medical.

M. Gravière, the sympathetic director of the theatre at Bordeaux, who has always lived in the midst of artists, and who has himself sung tenor, is persuaded that the great majority of singers often unconsciously adopt the costal method, which is the only one to be recommended.

M. L——, an amateur much sought after in drawing-rooms, and endowed with a pretty tenor voice, which he manages very well, defends the same ideas as we ourselves. Each time he fills an important *rôle*, that of Vincent or of José, for example, in " Mireille " and " Carmen," he has the habit of constricting his abdomen a little with a large belt ; he is then fatigued much less.

We have met with five other artists, who, at the theatre, have always taken the precaution of enrolling the abdomen with a band of flannel for the purpose of slightly compressing it ; by this means their voice is better sustained, and more resistant.

We may even speak of one of them—viz., M. Renaldi—who holds the position of second tenor in the Italian Company. This artist, while at the Conservatoire, was in the class of a master who made his pupils breathe abdominally. This method soon led to a general deterioration ; the breath became short, and the sounds of extreme feebleness, and the singer wished to renounce the theatre. But he modified his manner of breathing, and constructed for himself a mechanical belt which obliged him to contract the abdomen and to dilate the inferior part of the chest. M. Renaldi stated to us that his strength returned rapidly, that his thoracic circumference was considerably developed, and that he succeeded in holding a note for forty-five seconds.

Morell Mackenzie has also dwelt upon the good effects of a moderately tight belt. " The most casual observer must have noticed that when a fresh muscular effort has to be made, the abdominal walls are drawn in on inspiration. The diver who is going to plunge into the water, the warrior who is about to deliver a mighty blow, instinctively draw in and fix the abdominal walls. The Scriptural phrase of ' girding up the loins,' may be a figurative expression, having reference to this instinctive procedure, or may be an allusion to the use of the sash or belt so commonly employed in the East. These articles of dress of course intensify the flattening of the abdominal walls, and thus artificially assist in controlling the escape of breath."

Everybody knows, moreover, that belts are useful to runners and to persons who make great physical efforts. Among the Greeks, wrestlers made use of them until the thirty-fourth olympiad.

In singers it is easy to understand that a belt surrounding the inferior part of the abdomen, and not impeding the costal expansion, can counteract the weakness of the abdominal walls, and help the latter to support the weight of the viscera. Moreover, in presenting a more resistant fulcrum to these same viscera, and limiting their descent, it will diminish the work of the muscles of the abdominal walls, and will favour the elevation of the inferior ribs by the diaphragm, thus facilitating the accomplishment of the respiratory act according to the costal method.

We have now concluded the study of the different methods of respiration employed in singing, and we arrive at the conclusion that artists ought by preference to practise costal respiration, with slight depression of the inferior portion of the abdomen on inspiration :

1. Because it dilates the chest in its three diameters, transverse, vertical, and antero-

posterior, and permits the storing of a greater volume of air than is possible in the clavicular and abdominal methods ;

2. Because it favours the production of thoracic vibrations, and increases the power of the pectoral harmonics ;

3. Because it acts over the whole of the thoracic cavity, utilises the different forces of respiration, and divides the total work over a greater number of agents, whence there is greater resistance to fatigue ;

4. Because, thanks to the antagonism of the inspiratory and external expiratory muscles, it permits a graduation of the exit of the air and the economising of the wind ;

5. Because it is founded upon physiological laws according to which thoracic effort is produced ;

6. Because it is employed by the majority of singers, advised by the most renowned artists, and recommended by the old Italian masters, who have carried to such a high degree of perfection the art of singing.

CHAPTER X.

EDUCATION OF RESPIRATION.

Importance of good respiration in singing.—Characters
of inspiration and expiration in an experienced
artist.—It is necessary to commence respiratory
studies early.—Methodical exercises applied to
costal respiration.—Duration of exercises ; avoidance of fatigue.—Ordinary gymnastics increase
the respiratory power.

ARTISTIC respiration is to singing what
ordinary respiration is to life ; the one
and the other preside over the regular performance of the vital and vocal functions. A
man will enjoy good health only so long as
the respiratory act can be accomplished under
the best conditions. The artist, also, to
become an excellent singer, ought to be in
possession of a powerful bellows, with a
motor element which he can regulate perfectly.

" Proper management of the breath," says
Morell Mackenzie,* " is a fundamental con-

---

* *Loc. cit.*, First Edition.

dition of good singing, and however beautiful
the voice may be in itself, it can never be
used with artistic effect if the method of
respiration is faulty."

It is also necessary, by methodical education, commenced early and long continued,
by the use of well-chosen and frequently
repeated exercises, to correct vicious respiratory practices, to develop the natural gifts
of the artist, and to cause him to arrive at
that degree of perfection with which the
greatest singers know how to utilise their
respiration.

" Unfortunately," writes Crivelli,* "this important branch of the art of singing is almost
always neglected, either from the inexperience
of the master, or by reason of the negligence
of the singer. Very few singers make good
use of respiration, and often in endeavouring
to sing with expression, they succeed only in
making sounds which are disagreeable to the
ear, and in rendering themselves ridiculous
by their contortions."

We are not going so far as to say, with
certain authors, that this insufficiency of
study, so far as regards respiration, is the

* *Arte del canto.* London, s. d.

principal cause of the actual decadence of the vocal art ; but we recognise that many professors cause detriment to their pupils, either by inculcating false doctrines or by making a show of complete disinterestedness as to the different respiratory methods. These latter, more numerous than one would be tempted to believe, either from scepticism or ignorance, affect to maintain that it is indifferent for the singer to inspire or expire according to any particular method.

It is thus that Ponchard *père** writes : " No one has sung more than I. It is true that in my time music was not taught as scientific-ally as to-day. We sang with the means with which nature had endowed us, without troubling ourselves whether we breathed with the ribs or the diaphragm. And it is a singular thing that, in spite of our profound ignorance of the art of breathing, and of many other things, we sang well and for long with our poor natural voices, while since scientists have set themselves to fatigue voices, we hear speak only of ruined singers and lost voices."

We energetically protest against such pre-

* Burq, *De la gymnastique pulmonaire*. Paris, 1875.

tensions, which would lead to the negation of every system of education.

With rare exceptions, it is easy to recognise a subject who has submitted the muscular agents of respiration to exercises and methodical training. Observe a pupil at the beginning of his studies, and you will notice with what *maladresse* he puts his "bellows" in action. After having made a hurried, noisy, and incomplete inspiration, he allows the air to escape and waste to no purpose before commencing to sing. The sounds are not held for more than a few seconds, expiration is sudden and irregular, respiratory movements are frequent, from whence follows fatigue and rapid deterioration. On the contrary, in an accomplished singer, inspiration ought to be :—

1. *Calm.*—The introduction of the air is accomplished without violence and without roughness ; the chest is dilated in a regular fashion, without shocks or jerks, under pain of augmenting the muscular expenditure and provoking breathlessness ;

2. *Ample.*—The thorax assumes its greatest dimensions, in order to store up the largest amount of wind possible ;

3. *General.*—The amplification of the chest

is not limited to any one region ; all the muscular forces are utilised, from whence there
is a division of the work and diminution of
fatigue ;

4. *Silent.*—The column of air passes freely
across the larynx largely opened ; the vocal
cords are not put into vibration ; the inspiratory voice called "*hoquet dramatique*" is not
produced ; its hurtful consequences, tremor
and laryngeal catarrh, are no longer to be
dreaded.

After having inspired, the accomplished
singer maintains the air behind the glottis,
which is closed for an instant, in order to
avoid the loss of wind before the vocal cords
enter into vibration.   In different cases, and
according to the effect to be produced, the
sound is attacked without suddenness by a
slight movement of the edges of the glottis,
which opens suddenly, without jerk and without contraction ; or the note is emitted by a
vigorous shock similar to the action of the lips
in pronouncing the letter *p* energetically.
This is the famous "*coup de glotte*" of Garcia,
which it is necessary to employ with modera-
tion, because it exacts an increase of work
in the laryngeal organ ; it has, however, the

advantage of rendering more expressive, more vigorous, and more energetic, certain musical passages.

Lastly, the experienced artist regulates the exit of the air with perfect precision, according to his will ; in him expiration is at will :—

1. *Powerful* in great vocal declamation;

2. *Feeble* when he sings piano, pianissimo ;

3. *Prolonged* in musical phrases of long duration ;

4. *Equal* and regular in order to hold a note.

"The human voice," say MM. Lemaire and Lavoix, "ought to adapt itself to all the exigencies of the musical drama, and all the laws of declamation, even when these laws are not always of the purest vocal style. But how can it be the humble servant of him who directs it, how can it be at once light and powerful, to fly on the wings of a passionate *allegro*, or to follow the meanderings of a recitative with varied accents, or an expressive *largo*, if the singer has not been exercised early in all the difficulties of singing, if he has not learned from the commencement of his studies to perfectly manage the respiration, which one may almost call the motive power of the human voice ? "

It is essential that the pupil should learn to respire, from his earliest lessons, when the education of the muscles of respiration should be conducted at the same time as that of the muscles of the larynx, for these two muscular groups are far from being independent of one another in their phonatory functions ; we shall even see, in studying *vocal compensation*, that the height of the sound is due to the tension of the cords and to the pressure of the expired air, and that there is established a veritable co-ordination between the laryngeal and thoracic forces.

Is it necessary to await the complete development of the thorax before commencing the studies of pulmonary gymnastics, as some authors contend, under the fear of determining premature injury to young chests?   We believe, along with most professors, that it is necessary to occupy ourselves with respiration from infancy, with the precautions, of course, necessary to that age.

According to Morell Mackenzie,* " the first step in any system of instruction must therefore be to teach the pupil how and when to take the air into his lungs, and how to control

* *Loc. cit.* [*Vocal Gymnastics*], First Edition, p. 105.

and direct the outflow as he empties them. This is really one of the most difficult things in the whole art of singing ; but it must be mastered at whatever cost, for it is a vital point."

The same author remarks, as to the vocal training of children : " So far from injuring the general health, the teaching of singing in childhood is likely to prove highly beneficial, especially in cases in which there is a tendency to delicacy of the lungs. By the healthful exercise of these organs in singing, the chest is expanded, the muscles of respiration are strengthened, and the lungs themselves are made firmer and more elastic. The rare occurrence of pulmonary disease among singers is well known. Of course, it must be understood that the vocal exercises are to be strictly moderate, both as to quality and quantity—that is to say, the lessons must be very short, and at the most only the ten or twelve notes which form the average compass of a child's voice must be used. On no account must there be the least forcing or fatigue."*

All the work of the larynx ought to be suspended or reduced during the period of

* *Loc. cit.*, First Edition, p. 129.

breaking the voice ; that epoch of life can be
consecrated to the education of respiration.*

"During the breaking of the voice," says
Mandl,† "the raucous and hoarse voice is

---

* All authors are not, however, agreed upon this
point. For example, Morell Mackenzie thinks that,
with *due care*, the voice may be used in singing during
the period of breaking. Each case should be judged
on its merits; and while there are some voices which
might be ruined by singing through this period,
Mackenzie thinks that a "judicious teacher will have
no difficulty in deciding as to the best course to adopt
in any given instance." He remarks : " Unless the
larynx is much congested and the voice hoarse at the
period of change, I am strongly of opinion that vocal
training should be continued—of course, *within certain
limits—under competent supervision, and with due
precautions against overwork*" (*Hygiene of the Vocal
Organs*, Seventh Edition, p. 130). It is true that
Manuel Garcia is, among many others, opposed to
such a course, having himself lost his voice by this very
practice. It is therefore clear that there is a considerable
degree of risk in permitting a young person at this period
of physiological transition to continue singing, and, not-
withstanding the indisputable authority of Mackenzie, it
would seem wiser not to court accidents, by suspending
laryngeal work during the breaking of the voice, and to
occupy the time more profitably by the education of
respiration. The "competent supervision," and the "due
precautions," insisted upon by Mackenzie, are too often
absent from the control of the young musician.—TRANS.

† *Hygiene de la Voix*.

opposed to every serious exercise, which, moreover, would be dangerous, for it would hinder the normal development of the larynx, and might lead to a profound alteration or total loss of the voice. Professors of singing also should limit themselves to correcting the grosser defects of pronunciation or of emission, and directing the articulation."

This would also be, in our opinion, a favourable moment for exercises of respiration, and in general for exercises of vocal gymnastics.

These exercises should be conducted in a standing position ; the dorsal decubitus has, in fact, the inconvenience of impeding the movements of the ribs. The pupil should assume the position of a soldier, the body erect on the hips, the arms pendant, the hands joined.

" Placed erect," said Mannstein,* " the bust should be carried a little higher than in the position of ease ; the body would fall into position naturally, and this attitude would have the advantage of rendering the action of the diaphragm more free, and consequently of facilitating respiration."

The shoulders should be set back, and the chest should be advanced by raising the sternum.

* *Loc. cit.*

According to Mandl,* Monvoe (of Boston) made a special study of this displacement of the sternum ; independently of inspiration and expiration, this exercise is repeated thirty or forty times consecutively for three or four minutes, and several times a day.   At the end of some weeks the pupil easily succeeds in causing the thorax to assume the desired position as a matter of course.

It is necessary also to practise early to render oneself master of the movements of the abdominal muscles.   To this end M. Jean de Reszké recommends rapid contraction and relaxation of these muscles in their inferior third, practising the movement also a certain number of times consecutively, and several times a day.

These preliminary exercises having been properly executed, the pupil will pass to the following :—

He inspires slowly, deeply, and regularly, with an absolute immobility of the first ribs and the clavicles, raising and carrying outwards the middle and lower parts of the sternum, and of the costal apparatus, leaving the fold over the stomach to participate in the move-

* *Hygiène de la voix.*

ment of the elevation of the sternum and the amplification of the ribs, retracting slightly the umbilical and hypogastric part of the abdomen. Respiration is then maintained by means of the contraction of the inspiratory muscles, at first for three or four seconds, then progressively, after a few weeks up to twelve and thirteen seconds. Expiration is sudden and rapid.

The expiratory exercise which completes the preceding exercises consists, on the contrary, in inspiring rapidly after the method indicated, and making slow, gentle, and regular expirations, of a duration at first of a few seconds, reaching in the end its prolongation for as long as possible. The exit of the wind should be regulated by the muscles of respiration alone, without any intervention of the laryngeal muscles, and according to Garcia it is necessary to succeed in regulating the flow of air with so much gentleness that the flame of a lighted candle placed before the mouth ought not to oscillate.

Lastly, inspiratory and expiratory exercises are combined, and the pupil will experience no difficulty in doing so when he will have learned to execute either separately.

It is essential to correct at once bad habits of respiration.

To persons who raise their shoulders in inspiring, Mandl recommends "the crossing of the arms as high as possible, in a seated position over the back of a chair." The shoulders are thus rendered immovable, and clavicular respiration impossible; the same result may be arrived at by pressing the sides of the neck between the arms of a chair, or in the corner of a couch, or by any other similar means.

To pupils who during inspiration protrude the inferior portion of the abdomen, it is necessary to recommend the use of a large belt which moderately compresses the abdomen in its sub-umbilical portion.

There is scarcely any need to say that thoracic dilatation ought never to be impeded by any constrictive clothing, and that women, in order properly to practise the costal type, will be obliged to renounce tight corsets, which impede the play of the diaphragm and the expansion of the lower ribs.

Lablache * and Manuel Garcia † agree that

Méthode complète de chant. Paris.

† *Traité complet de l'art du chant.* Paris ; Heugel, 1840.

the respiratory exercises ought to be made without voicing ; on the contrary, Panofka, * Lemaire, and Lavoix, think that this method serves only to fatigue the lungs, without any profit to the singer. We cannot agree with this latter opinion ; we believe that every exercise having for its aim the development and the control of the muscles of respiration will produce the same effect if it is performed without any vocalisation. Moreover, the pupil, when not singing, is obliged to leave the glottis open, and the contraction of the laryngeal muscles cannot contribute to the retarding of the exit of air ; the expiratory movement is under the sole dependence of the muscular powers of respiration.

Respiratory studies can be made at any hour of the day, but they should be performed by preference in the morning while fasting, or before a meal, when the stomach contains no food, and digestion is not yet proceeding.

In order to derive the greatest benefit from these respiratory exercises, it is indispensable not to repeat them and prolong them until fatigue occurs. To exaggerate the work, to make it pass beyond certain limits, will rapidly

* *L'Art de Chanter.* Paris : Brandus.

lead to impairment of the respiratory powers, will lead to loss of elasticity of the pulmonary tissue, and will occasion, on the part of the larynx, troubles in the vascularisation of the mucous membrane, and in the mobility of muscles.   This pathological condition would have the harmful consequence of necessitating a rest of long duration, and also of assiduous care; the definitive loss of the voice might even result.

Young people in particular should be put upon their guard against the dangers that they run when, in singing, they abuse their motive force, giving too great intensity to sounds, holding them too long, and thus forcing their respiration.   Boisquel* expresses himself thus upon this point :—

" The air expands the numerous fibres of the lungs, which are too young and too feeble to support this fatigue.   At twenty years of age, respiration is made with noise, and at twenty-five there is a marked deterioration in the voice.   Young chests demand the greatest management ; and in order that the exit of air may be passable, it is necessary not to seek to '*filer les sons*.' †

* *Essai sur l'art du comédien chanteur.*   Paris, 1812.
† The " *mezza di voce.*"

" This should only be done when the nubile age. has given to the lungs their necessary solidity.   The voice would acquire very much more force, and more energy, and would be more pure and more harmonious."

Moreover, all exercises leading to the production of fatigue ought to be avoided in the physical exercises of which we have just spoken, and which are recommended by all authors in order to strengthen the muscles of respiration.

All the elementary practices of the ordinary gymnasium (movements of the arms backwards and forwards, dumb-bells, elastic belts, parallel bars, etc.) are useful to the singer, by causing him to throw into function the muscles which are inserted on the trunk and upper limbs.

" Walking and pedestrian exercises," said Mandl, "are the most advantageous of all exercises for the organs of respiration, especially simple walking, much more than jumping, running, hunting, dancing, etc. *Fencing*, specially, by exercising alternately the two sides, is very useful in developing the muscles of the thorax, without speaking of the other advantages which it gives, such as suppleness, grace, etc. *Swimming* is also an exercise very favourable to the development and amplification of the thoracic cavity ; it gives tone and energy to the muscles employed. *Rowing* develops in a very advantageous manner the amplitude of the chest and the muscular strength of the arms."

We have already said that Chassagne and Dally have undertaken researches upon the gymnasts of the school of Joinville, and have demonstrated after five months of training a sensible increase in the bi-mammary thoracic circumference.

From all these facts it is rational to conclude that it is indispensable for the singer to submit the muscles of respiration to methodical exercises, in order to increase his thoracic capacity, to prolong the duration of the expiratory movement, and to regulate the exit of air at his will.

CHAPTER XI.

HYGIENE OF RESPIRATION.

Necessity of good hygiene.—Influence of vitiated, damp, or dry air.—Action of dust: nasal inspiration.—Dwellings.—Aspect of apartments, heating, lighting, clothing: flannel, silk, corset, braces, belts.—Nitrogenous and carbonaceous foods: spirits, coffee.—Hours of meals.—Muscular exercises.

AFTER having glanced at artistic respiration from the educational point of view, it becomes necessary to inquire under what conditions the singer should be placed in order to preserve to the motor of the vocal machine the power and regularity which it has acquired. "Take care of your lungs, and the voice will take care of itself," writes Lennox Browne,* paraphrasing an old proverb; and his long experience has led him to the conclusion that, in many cases, vocal troubles are due to defective respiration. That is to say, it is of the first necessity

* *Loc. cit*

148

for the singer to be freed from baneful
influences, which may impede the regular
course of the pulmonary air-blast, whether
these arise from the world around him or
from his own organism. We therefore believe
it useful to indicate here some hygienic principles which bear particularly upon respiration,
and to examine the modifications which this
function may undergo, under the influence of
various surroundings, dwellings, clothing,
food, etc.

Many interesting questions arise in the
study of respiration in its relationship to the
atmospheric air. First, the air which the
singer breathes ought always to be of great
purity ; that is to say, it ought to contain four
parts of nitrogen, one part of oxygen, and
only traces of carbonic acid and watery
vapour. In confined spaces, in badly ventilated rooms, overheated and crowded with
people, the proportion of oxygen diminishes,
while that of carbonic acid increases. Every
one knows the fatigue experienced by remaining in such surroundings ; the face becomes
congested, and headache follows. Oxygen,
necessary to the pulmonary exchange, being
diminished, the respiratory movements

become more frequent, inspiration is consequently less ample, and expiration shorter.
It is therefore necessary to advise artists to
avoid concert-rooms and *salons* of limited
space, and badly ventilated, where they are
exposed to the loss of part of their vocal
powers. An overheated atmosphere is just
as prejudicial to the singer.

" When it is too hot," says Mandl,* " respiration is retarded, and the individual stifles ;
the voice is feeble, dragging, and failing in all
brilliancy."

But the great enemy of the bronchial tubes
is cold and wet air, which especially exercises
its hurtful effects upon persons whose habit it
is to breathe through the mouth. The cavity
of the mouth serves both to receive food and
to articulate sound ; the natural passage of
the air is through the nasal fossæ, which are
designed for the heating and drying of the
air before it penetrates the lungs.

From the external wall of each nasal
passage depend three small osseous and
curved structures, which, along with the
septum of the nose itself, are covered with
erectile tissue, which increases in volume, or

* *Hygiène de la voix parlée et chantée.*

expands, by the filling of large blood spaces within it, and under the control of the nervous system, in such a manner that a considerable quantity of blood is enclosed in a comparatively limited space. The air, circulating in contact with this tissue, extracts heat from it, and becomes of a temperature approaching that of the body when it traverses the bronchial tubes.

"The air," says Morell Mackenzie,* "ought always to pass through its natural canal, the nose; the mouth is to be employed only as an auxiliary passage, when absolutely necessary," when, for example, musical phrases are very short, and exact rapid inspirations. The action of cold air upon the broncho-tracheal mucous membrane determines congestive attacks and creates inflammatory conditions of this membrane.

Nasal inspiration has another advantage which ought to be mentioned; viz., that of partly ridding the air of dust and inorganic and organic particles which it contains. After a night at a ball, after certain railway journeys, or several hours' walking in manufacturing towns, most persons reject blackish mucus from

* *Loc. cit.*

the nasal fossæ or the naso-pharynx ; this consists of dust which the nasal mucous membrane has arrested in its passages, and which has thus been prevented from penetrating into the bronchial tubes, which however are only incompletely protected, and which end in being irritated if the singer is frequently exposed to the influence of this dust.

In certain countries, England in particular, in order to combat the inconveniences of cold, moist, and dusty air, the use of *respirators* is pretty general.* These are small apparatuses, often made of hardened felt, which when heated can be moulded to the face. The central part of their structure, corresponding to the buccal and nasal openings, is made of a thin layer of cotton wool, which acts in the manner of a filter for hurtful particles, at the same time drying and warming the inspired air. These respirators are also capable of opposing a barrier to the infectious germs which penetrate into the economy by the air-passages.

It is especially a sudden change in tem-

* The reader will doubtless smile at this very Gallic conception of the rigours of the English climate. The climate of London is little, if any, worse than that of Paris.—TRANSLATOR.

perature of the surroundings which the singer must dread ; thus, in severe cold he ought not to go out of a very hot room into the street without the greatest precaution, under risk of contracting a chill or an inflammation of the bronchial mucous membrane.

On those days when an artist will have to interpret an important part, to produce a great vocal effort, he should remain indoors, and should abstain from all walking exercise, if the atmosphere is charged with electricity, or if a hot, dry wind prevails, for these climatic conditions will generally have a baneful influence upon the respiration, and produce a condition of depression which causes the voice to temporarily lose its power and brilliancy.

"Volatile substances," said Mandl, "scarcely act directly upon the organs of voice, but they sometimes exert an indirect influence by acting upon the nervous system. Migraines, vertigos, nauseas, giddiness, have been observed in women of nervous temperament who remain in a room full of flowers." (*See* Appendix.)

We shall see later on that certain bodies, in the form of powders, and certain odours, can produce an impression upon the pituitary mucous membrane of subjects predisposed, to the point of provoking erection of the cavernous tissue of the nose, and determining a reflex phenomenon which is evidenced by a veritable dyspnœic crisis, or by slight depression of the respiratory strength. This is a danger which it is necessary to indicate to singers who are rheumatic, or irritable, and especially to those born of asthmatic parents.

In the choice of a residence or lodging the artist should pay attention also to certain hygienic principles. During fine weather, if possible, he should live in the country by preference, the pure air of which is very beneficial to the respiratory organs ; the tonic and vivifying atmosphere of the mountains is especially to be recommended ; on the contrary, during winter the streets of towns are more suitable, less humid, and the collection together of a number of houses diminishes the intemperateness of bad weather. A dwelling should not be newly constructed, it should be in a dry and sunny spot : the apartment should have a good aspect, and be protected from cold winds ; it should be rather high up, and the rooms should be spacious, and with sufficient openings to permit of easy and rapid ventilation. The ceilings should be high, and it is essential that respiration may not suffer from the excess of carbonic acid which is found in the air of small rooms. The walls should not be covered with hangings, nor the floor with carpets, since the voice then loses in sonority, and the singer, in order to overcome this, has to force his sounds and exaggerate his expiratory pressure, until fatigue follows as a matter of course.

Stoves, when used for the heating of rooms, have the drawbacks of emitting disagreeable odours, and drying the air too much, which ought always to contain a certain quantity of watery vapour.

Ordinary stoves produce an oppressive heat, which frequently gives rise to headaches. We prefer the ordinary fireplace, in spite of the loss of heat which results ; wood and coke * are preferable to coal, which produces smoke and gases, similarly hurtful to the organs of respiration.

For lighting, nothing is superior to the

* In the ordinary English fireplaces, coke would be quite out of the question, being both difficult to burn, and producing extremely noxious fumes.—TRANSLATOR.

electric light ; the purified oils of colza and petroleum may also be used, but it is necessary to dispense with gas, in spite of its great convenience, for it converts a considerable amount of the atmospheric air into carbonic acid gas, and greatly increases the temperature of the ambient medium. " I know nothing," says Mandl,* " more contrary to hygiene than the small apartments of artists, where the latter have to dress and to suffocate between two gas jets, the source of a stifling heat, and an atmosphere less and less respirable. The windows have then to be opened, and the individual is exposed to draughts, or else the singer goes out from this stuffy atmosphere to appear upon a stage, often icy in temperature, especially in winter. Is it astonishing that such conditions should be a frequent cause of inflammatory affections of the respiratory passages or of the larynx ? "

Nowadays most theatres are lighted with electricity ; only in small towns do we meet with gas and with deplorable conditions, which should be got rid of at any price.

The question of *clothing* is interesting to

* *Loc cit.*

study, if we consider it in relation to the
respiration of the singer. In ordinary life
the artist has no special rules to follow,
provided that he considers the weather and
the season ; during winter, it is well to have
woollen clothing, which better preserves the
heat of the body, and to invest the skin with
flannel, which favours the cutaneous functions,
imbibes the perspiration, and, preventing its
rapid evaporation, wards off chills.

On rainy days, overcoats of impermeable
stuffs are not to be despised, and the same
may be said of rubber shoes, which quite
protect the feet against wet and cold, such
frequent causes of tracheo-bronchitis ; but
the use of these impermeable materials ought
to be only temporary, for they condense the
internal transpiration, and the damp which
they cause to accumulate around the skin
causes the latter to be more susceptible to
variations of temperature.

Singers are obliged, at the theatre, to wear
the most varied costumes, but these should
never be heavy, or so worn as to impede
the movements of the thorax ; if on the stage
the artist is clothed in a costume too hot or
too light, he ought to take special precautions

when retiring from the stage behind the scenes or into his dressing-room.

All authors who have occupied themselves with vocal hygiene have dwelt upon the respiratory insufficiency caused by the corset; some have formally proscribed its use ; others are content with prohibiting this article of clothing in its most pernicious forms.

Morell Mackenzie * remarks : " As for tight lacing, where the pressure is severe enough actually to deform bones and displace organs, and where the corset resembles a surgical apparatus for fixing the ribs, it is a species of stupidity for which hardly a parallel can be found even among the innumerable follies of civilised life. . . . A well-made woman should not require stays ; and where some support is needed, the corset should be made of elastic material, yielding readily to the natural movements of the trunk, with just enough whalebone to give it firmness. Steels are an abomination which should be left to the foolish virgins whose devotion to fashion makes them willing to rival the Fakîr in self-martyrdom. Rigid stays, in short, should be relegated to the museums, to be exhibited

* *Loc. cit.*, p. 142.

side by side with the Collar, the Boot, the Maiden, and other mediæval instruments of torture."

Bernard Roth,* who has made a complete study of the subject, writes : " The lower ribs, which are least supported in front, are precisely those which are influenced by anything tight about the waist ; thus, close-fitting, unyielding *stays*, as generally worn, gradually compress the yielding lower ribs more and more, till their anterior extremities, instead of being far apart, meet almost, or quite, in the middle line. This deformity occurs so gradually during years of growth that the wearer is generally quite unconscious of having disfigured herself. . . . This pressing inward of the ribs, which become in time permanently deformed, causes necessarily a very great diminution in the size of the chest and abdominal cavities."

À propos of the difference of the respiratory type in the male and female sex in ordinary life, we have already maintained (p. 21) that the clavicular method is characteristic of the female sex, not on account of the phenomena

* *Dress : its Sanitary Aspect.* London : Churchill, 1880.

of gestation, as was generally supposed, but
from the continual usage of the corset for
many generations. We have quoted the ex-

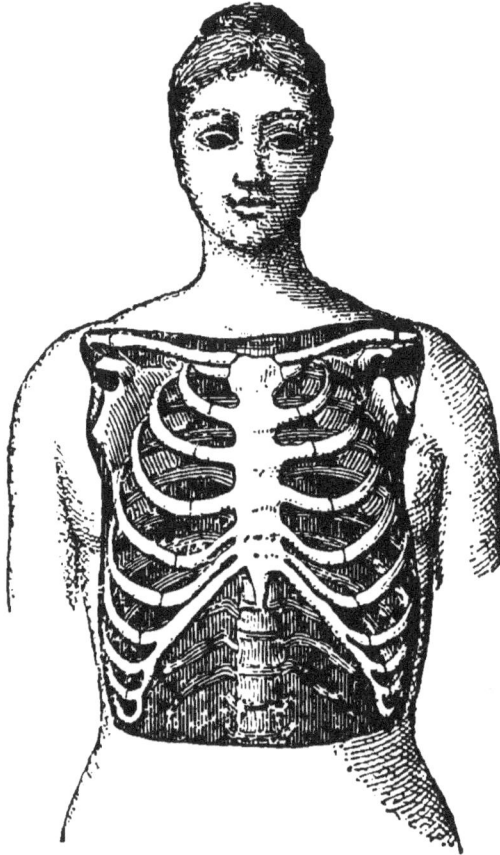

FIG. 8.

periments of two American physicians, which
establish the fact that in uncivilised Indian
women, who wear no constrictive clothing,
respiration is not conducted according to the

clavicular method, but just as in man, upon the abdominal type.

It is therefore to the corset that we must attribute the vitiation of the respiratory

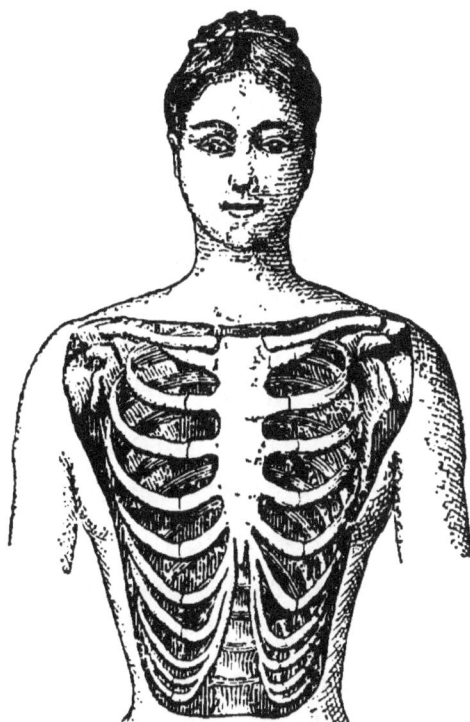

FIG. 9.—Deformity of chest through wearing of corsets. (After Lennox Browne.)

method in the weaker sex, the special deformity of the chest found in certain individuals, and the lowering of the vital capacity in all those who compress the figure.

Lennox Browne* has undertaken researches

* *Voice, Song, and Speech*, Twelfth Edition, p. 97.

upon this latter point with the spirometer ;
and this instrument has furnished him in the
majority of cases with such indications that
he feels justified in drawing the conclusion
that the volume of air expired varies by
nearly a third, more or less, according as the
thorax is free or imprisoned in a corset of
inflexible structure.

"A young lady," says he, "who by her
height should, according to Hutchinson's
tables, breathe 145 cubic inches, was able with
difficulty to inhale 100 ; but on removal of
her stays at once and with ease blew 140
cubic inches into the spirometer. Another
lady, less than 5 feet high, should have
breathed about 120 cubic inches. Before the
removal of her corsets she managed, after
several violent efforts, to breathe 75 inches
only, but afterwards at the first attempt she
breathed 108 inches. She discontinued the
use of these stays, and took to others without whalebone or steel, and continued to
maintain this gain in her chest expansion."

We have repeated these experiments under
the same conditions in a large number of
women, and the volumetric measurements
obtained with our apparatus demonstrate that

the respiratory loss due to the action of the corset may vary between 200 to 1100 cubic centimètres ; the more rigid and tight the clothing, the more is the movement of thoracic expansion interfered with.

These various considerations should lead us to pronounce a formal interdiction of the corset ; we scarcely dare to do so, from the fear of not being listened to ; but we may at least go so far as to advise ladies who sing to use a corset as supple and ample as the exigencies of fashion permit.

The upholders of diaphragmatic respiration recommend the employment of braces instead of a belt, which, by compressing the abdomen, impedes the descent of the diaphragm. We have, on the contrary, maintained that a belt, moderately tight, below the ribs, is of service to the singer who employs the costal method of respiration, and that it furnishes a point of assistance to the abdominal viscera, and thus facilitates the elevation of the ribs by the diaphragm.

Braces have the advantage, by reason of the pressure which they exert upon the clavicle, of diminishing the tendency to raise the shoulders which some artists possess.

Ought the neck to be exposed, or protected by wraps and mufflers? We believe that the habit of covering the neck renders this part of the body more subject to suffer impressions of cold and variations of temperature; but we recognise the fact that many attacks of laryngitis, tracheitis, or bronchitis, will be avoided if persons susceptible to these complaints take the precaution of enveloping this part with a silk handkerchief, in damp weather, when they go out of a very hot room.

If we now inquire what ought to be the dietary *régime* of a singer, we may remark that it is difficult enough to lay down any general rules or advice applicable to everybody.

Each person should be guided by his own experience in determining, as to articles of diet, what is good and what is harmful.

As Morell Mackenzie remarks : * " Let a man eat to the satisfaction of his natural appetite what his palate craves and his stomach does not kick against ; an adult has, as a rule, been taught what his aliment should

* *Hygiene of the Vocal Organs*, Seventh Edition, p. 137.

be by that most practical physician—experience.   Let him take his meals at regular
intervals, and chew his food properly, and
he may laugh at the highly rarefied *menus*
dictated by the framers of dietetic decalogues."

It is well to remark that in singers the
amplitude and frequency of the respiratory
movements, and default of physical exercise
will necessitate the ingestion of a more than
usually large proportion of carbonaceous food.
It is well known that food is divided into two
large classes : *nitrogenous*, nutritive, and repa-
rative, serving for the regeneration of tissues
(meat, cheese, eggs, milk); *carbo-hydrates*, heat-
forming, respiratory, which furnish carbonic
acid exhaled by the lungs and skin, and the
principal source of the heat formation of the
body (fats, oils, sugar, vegetables, fruits). The
latter ought to predominate in the diet of a
singer who does not take great physical
exercise.

Before undertaking any vocal effort, sustained and fatiguing in character, the singer
ought to abstain from food not easy of digestion.   The meal should not be too hearty, and
ought to be taken three or four hours before
appearing upon the stage.   It is easily under-

stood that it is indispensable not to distend
the stomach with too much food, especially
when this is difficult of digestion, or tends to
produce much gas ; the volume and weight of
the stomach and of the intestinal mass, prevent the diaphragm from free movement, and
determine respiratory weakness, which is most
pronounced in those singers who employ the
abdominal type.   Most of the artists of the
Opéra and *Opéra comique* are in the habit of
not dining at all on the days of their appearance ; they take a slight collation at three or
four o'clock in the afternoon, and supper at
night, after leaving the theatre.

The moderate use of coffee, tea, or spirits,
cannot be reprehensible ; these in small doses
stimulate digestion ; but if they are abused
the general circulation is accelerated, and
respiration is both more frequent and deeper.
We have no need here to refer to the disorders
of the system produced by alcoholism.

Certain individuals can smoke with impunity
after a meal ; nevertheless, we do not advise
artists to follow their example, because to-
bacco, besides determining pharyngo-laryngi-
tis, momentarily produces an excitation of
the nervous system, which is manifested in

acceleration of the beating of the heart and by rapid and irregular respiratory movements.

Before terminating this short review of the alimentary hygiene, let us impress upon ladies the necessity of attending to their intestinal functions, and combating that so frequent error of the sex, constipation, by the employment of articles of diet of a laxative character, green vegetables, compôtes of fruit, honey, etc. Individuals who breathe according to the costal method, retracting the lower part of the abdomen, should especially guard against this sluggishness of the bowels ; the volume of the descending colon of the rectum being exaggerated, the retraction of the abdomen becomes difficult.

Activity of the skin should be encouraged by baths, douches, frictions, etc., since if the cutaneous exhalation is badly performed, that of the lungs is increased, and the respiratory mucous membrane becomes more susceptible and more easily congested.

Muscular exercises of the arms and limbs are useful to the singer ; they also develop, as we have already said, the respiratory powers, they assist digestion and nutrition, and contribute to the maintenance of the general health.

But the work of the agents of locomotion ought to be limited, and not to be pushed to the point of fatigue or tiredness, which would have a hurtful effect upon the thoracic muscles.

Lastly, late nights and immoderate pleasures are very prejudicial to artists, by lowering the nervous system and enfeebling the organism, excess leading to a depression of the respiratory apparatus.

CHAPTER XII.

RELATION BETWEEN THE MOTOR ELEMENT AND THE VIBRATING ELEMENT OF PHO-NATION.

Height of a sound.—*Rôle* of aërial pressure in laryngeal intonation. — Interdependence of the muscular agents of respiration and those of the larynx.— Vocal compensation. — Respiratory insufficiency robs the voice of its freshness, purity, agility, and extent.—Laryngeal congestions.—Acute laryngitis : chronic laryngitis of the same origin.

UP to now we have limited ourselves to establishing that a respiration powerful and easily controlled allows the singer to control the intensity of the voice, to measure the duration of sounds, and to graduate musical phrases. But there is another important *rôle* devolving upon the respiratory function, viz., that of contributing to the fixing of the height of sounds, and of taking part in that complex act which physiologists have studied under the name of *vocal compensation*, and to which we are now about to devote some words.

The laws of acoustics teach us that the height of a sound depends upon the number of vibrations executed by the sonorous body in a second, and that in a cord the number of vibrations varies in inverse ratio to its length, and its diameter, proportionally to the square root of its tension—inversely as the square root of its density.

Seeing the small dimensions of the glottis one of these four factors has such a preponderating value that the three others may be regarded as negligible quantities. Tension alone is the cardinal agent of modulation of the voice. But this tension is not the exclusive result of the contraction of the laryngeal muscles, as was formerly supposed, and as is maintained yet by some authors. It results likewise from the pressure of the expired air. This view has been defended by Ferrein (1741), Liscovius (1814), Müller (1845). In more recent times Lermoyez (1886) has adopted this teaching, which Battaille in 1861 had attempted in vain to rescue from oblivion.

Müller,* who made numerous experiments

* *Manuel de Physiologie.* French translation, by Jourdan. 1845.

upon the larynx of the cadaver, recognised that—

" With equal tension of the vocal cords, obtained by a weight, the greatest possible force of the air-blast raises the sound nearly a fifth, or even more, which indicates two processes in the production of the same sound ; a gentle air-blast with a given tension of the vocal cords, or a stronger air-blast with less tension. When the maximum of tension with which the vocal cords give the most acute sound possible is attained by a tranquil air-blast, we may yet, by employing a stronger air-blast, cause the emission of some sounds still more acute or shrill. Experiment upon ourselves demonstrates the same fact."

Artists, without occupying themselves with science, and by pure instinct, indeed, make use of these augmentations or diminutions of respiratory pressure in order to arrive at vocal results otherwise impossible of attainment. When they have reached the highest limits of their voices, and their muscles, contracted to the fullest extent, can give them no further assistance, they call to aid a stronger air-blast, and then succeed in emitting notes which muscular action alone would be powerless to produce. This is how "robust tenors" eject in full voice the chest *ut*, and deep basses, on the contrary, emit such feeble sounds in order to descend to the deepest notes.

Lermoyez,[*] who also has made cadaveric researches, arrives at the following conclusions:—"Classical treatises do not sufficiently insist upon the very important *rôle* which aërial pressure plays in the laryngeal determination ; when we study the formation of notes, we have not only to take into account the degree of muscular contraction which corresponds to a given pitch, but to consider at least as much the exact pressure of the air expired at this moment. We cannot emit any note without a certain degree of respiratory pressure, and this pressure alone produces a degree of glottic tension, which is superadded to the tension already produced by muscular action, so that every vocal pitch results from the sum of these two tensions. Instinctively or from education we obtain this addition of force with an exactitude so well combined that their sum is always what we wish, without, however, our knowing exactly how much of this muscular tension is

* *Étude expérimentale sur la phonation.* 1886.

attributable to muscular action and how much to aërial pressure."

We may add that the passive tension of the vocal cords by the confined air gives place to an enlargement of the glottic opening, so that certain authors have imagined in this fact they have found the explanation of vocal compensation. If, according to them, a singer can emit a note with more or less intensity, without modifying its pitch, it is due to the fact that the greater energy of the current of air is neutralised by a larger opening of the glottis, which, in dilating, offers less resistance to the exit of the air, and proportionally attenuates the pressure.

We prefer to adopt the opinion of Lermoyez, who interprets the mechanism of vocal compensation in another fashion, admitting that according as passive tension increases, the active tension diminishes from the progressively diminished contraction of the tensor muscles of the vocal cords.

In recalling these physiological facts, we have merely had the desire of directing the attention to the functional bonds which unite, in singing, the action of the laryngeal and thoracic muscles. These agents can replace one another, or assist each other in their work in such a fashion that when the activity of one is enfeebled, an excess of expenditure is thrown upon the others. Let the respiratory pressure be lowered, and the muscles of the larynx must contract with greater energy, become overworked, and consequently rapidly fatigued. The same inconveniences will occur when the vital capacity is diminished, the latter always following the oscillations of respiratory pressure.

Réné, who has experimented much with the spirometer, writes : * " The strength of inspiration and expiration is in relation with the functional activity of the lung. When the curve of vital capacity is lowered, the line representing the curve of the strength of inspiration and expiration is equally lowered. The two curves which indicate the pressure and the volume are nearly constantly parallel." We may therefore consider as equivalent the expressions : volume, strength, pressure, of the air expired, and we may employ one term for the other.

Let us now examine what laryngeal troubles may result from respiratory insufficiency.

* *Gaz. des Hopitaux.* 1880.

We have nothing to do with true dyspnœa, oppression, stifling, since these morbid conditions quite debar the practice of singing ; we merely have in sight those slight respiratory modifications which are scarcely revealed, except by the spirometer, or by pneumographic instruments.

Let us take the case of a singer whose respiration has become unconsciously sluggish, or less ample. This person, in order to produce the same vocal effects as formerly, has to exact increased work of his thoracic or laryngeal muscles. In the first case, the sounds may be emitted with just as much intensity, the duration of the musical phrases may be as long, high notes as easy as before ; but, in order to attain this, there is an exaggerated expenditure of strength, which is not long in leading to fatigue of the organs of respiration, and consecutive feebleness of the voice. Then the singer experiences trouble in holding sounds, the respiratory movements, less deep in extent, are more frequent, and the voice loses its amplitude and power ; a feeling of uneasiness, trouble, and weight, is felt in the chest. Sometimes even discomfort, painful points, or trembling movements are perceived at the moment of muscular contraction.

In a former work * we have instanced cases of this kind controlled by the spirometer—among others, that of an eminent artist of the opera who could no longer sing the "Rameaux" of Faure, because in the phrase "Celui qui vient sauver le monde" he could not hold the note on the word "monde" so long as he was in the habit of doing. The cure of a nasal affection, which had caused a diminution in the wind, restored to the illustrious baritone all his former vocal power.

Let us now pass to the second class of case, in which, the vital capacity being diminished, the larynx is overtaxed. The singer soon loses the freshness and the purity of his voice. The laryngeal muscles, submitted to exaggerated work, become sluggish, and execute their contractions with less regularity and precision ; they are less prompt to obey the will, and have no longer the same vigour and suppleness. Their movements are less accurate and delicate. The voice is no longer so flexible and agile as formerly, and vocalisation fails in grace and lightness. The

* *Réchcrches spirométriques.* Paris : Doin, 1890.

artist can no longer use the *mezza di voce*, high notes are emitted only with difficulty, and the voice may be even lowered by one or two tones.

We have known a great cantatrice, endowed with a marvellous dramatic soprano voice, who left the theatre because she could no longer reach the *si*^{4}, the *si*^{4} bemol, the *la*^{4}, and especially because it was impossible for her to use the *mezza di voce*, in which she had formerly excelled.   These troubles were caused by a respiratory insufficiency, of reflex origin.

Tremors may equally well proceed from incomplete respiration; the muscles of the larynx, under the influence of immoderate efforts, get the habit of contracting in jerks, and end by being removed entirely from the will.   " We have an exact idea of the condition," says Battaille,* " in comparing them to the muscular tremors which generally follow all prolonged work, as, for example, the holding at arms' length of a heavy weight."

Laryngeal troubles are revealed sometimes

* *De l'enseignement du chant.*   Paris: Masson, 1863.

by the numerous "couacs" which the singer interjects into acute chest notes, due to the sudden and involuntary passage from one register to another, which indicates that the artist is no longer in full possession of his vocal instrument.

These vocal manifestations occur generally without any morbid appearances of the laryngeal mucous membrane, but there are cases in which the overtaxing this organ, from lowering of the vital capacity, engender local disorders appreciable with the laryngoscope ; and this is the primary cause of the congestive attacks so frequently observed in singers. We then see fugitive congestions following upon moderate vocal effort, or after a short stay in dry atmosphere, slight cooling, the use of a few cigarettes, indeed after any of those influences to which the singer used formerly to offer great resistance. The blood reaches the arterioles and capillaries of the laryngeal mucous membrane under greater pressure, and the vascular walls are dilated. The vessels having become larger receive more blood, and a congestive condition is reached. But there are not yet any troubles in nutrition, the cellular elements do not participate in the irritation, and the phenomena do not attain the degree which constitutes inflammation.

We have studied elsewhere* these fluxions of the vocal mucous membrane, and have maintained that these congestive phenomena were essentially fugitive, disappearing at the end of a few hours, without leaving any trace of their presence. We have indicated as symptoms which are detected by the laryngoscope, redness and swelling of the mucous membrane. The injection, in the cases which interest us, is generally diffuse and generalised, it invades the whole larynx, being sometimes more marked over the region of the ventricular bands, sometimes extending to the mucous membrane of the pharynx and trachea. We have, then, to do with pharyngo-laryngeal or tracheo-laryngeal congestions. The swelling is never pronounced in character, especially over the true vocal cords, where the mucous membrane adheres intimately to the thyro-arytenoid ligament ; tumefaction rather occupies the upper portion of the larynx, the ventricular bands, the posterior

* *Étude sur les fluxions de la muqueuse laryngée. Revue de Laryngologie*, 1884.

commissure, the arytenoid region, and the ary-epiglottic ligaments, places where the mucous membrane is united to the subjacent layers by a loose and abundant cellular tissue, so that vascular dilatation and serous transudation are more easy.

Besides redness and swelling, the laryngeal mirror shows in some subjects a deficiency in the approximation of the vocal cords. These, instead of meeting during phonation, as in normal voice production, leave a small ellipsoid space in the middle part of the glottis; the free edges of the cords no longer have a parallel direction, but form a concave line.

We have, then, a bilateral paralysis of the tensor muscles of the cords, due to concomitant hyperæmia of the nerve filaments supplying these muscles. The akinesis may, however, be unilateral.

Subjective symptoms are indicated by disagreeable sensations, sometimes painful, which the patient feels behind the thyroid cartilage, discomfort, dryness, tickling or pricking, heat or burning sensations, which are always more acute in persons of neurotic constitution.

Cough is absent, in slight forms, or is dry, short, small, and resembling a frequent "hem." On the contrary, when the fluxion is intense and predominates over the arytenoid region, when the reflex excitability of the mucous membrane is heightened, the cough becomes incessant, spasmodic, and of raucous and deep tone.

The alterations of the voice also vary according to the patient, and the degree and localisation of the congestive phenomena ; sometimes the notes are dulled only in the demi-tone, but oftener there is hoarseness. Aphonia characterises complicated cases of bilateral paralysis.

After appearing a certain number of times, these congestive attacks become inflammatory if the singer is still subject to the same hurtful influences ; nutritive troubles are then produced in the tissues ; each attack is more tenacious, and lasts some days. Laryngoscopically, the redness and tumefaction are more marked, and we may even find small ulcerations upon the mucous membrane ; the cough is not always dry, and after its first period it becomes accompanied by slight expectoration. The symptoms of acute laryngitis are too well known to require us to dwell further upon them.

The repetition of inflammatory attacks ends in determining a chronic catarrhal condition of the mucous membrane; this becomes vascular, its connective tissue hyperplastic, and its glands hypertrophied. With the laryngo-scopic mirror the vocal cords are seen to be smooth, grey, thick ; the free edges are some-times unequal, and present small nodules. The voice loses its timbre, brightness, and purity ; muffled in ordinary language, it is rough upon the least effort. When chronic laryngitis has reached this degree, there is no longer any possibility of singing, and the artistic future is gravely compromised.

What therapeutic means should be adopted for these laryngeal conditions? First, and principally, at the first attacks an endeavour should be made to ascertain the cause which leads to the diminution of the vital capacity, and which provokes enfeeblement of the motor power, and to obtain the disappearance of the genetic conditions which we shall shortly indicate.

In congestions of the larynx, we advise inhalations and sprays of emollient and

slightly astringent substances, compresses
round the neck, a saline purgative, sinapisms
to the extremities, a potion of aconite, and
applications to the larynx of a feeble solution
of chloride of zinc.

In acute laryngitis we prescribe hot drinks,
vapour baths, tepid sprays with infusion of
coca leaves, revulsives, and derivatives; we
administer internally balsams, or benzoate of
soda ; and locally we give the preference to
medication with iodine or menthol solutions.

In chronic laryngitis, it is especially necessary to give carbolic sprays, swabbings of
nitrate of silver, and treatment at thermal
stations.

In cases of paralysis we ought to employ
electricity.

At acute periods, absolute rest of the vocal
organs must be recommended ; nothing being
more prejudicial to the voice than to sing
when the laryngeal mucous membrane is the
seat of a congestive or inflammatory attack.

CHAPTER XIII.

ETIOLOGICAL CONDITIONS PROVOKING LOWERING OF THE VITAL CAPACITY.

Use of the spirometric indications.—Respiratory feebleness due to overwork.—Change of method.—Nasal affections ; obstruction, reflex phenomena.—Hypertrophy of the palatine or lingual tonsils ; chronic pharyngitis.—Emphysema and pulmonary tuberculosis in their beginnings. —Gastralgias, flatulent dyspepsia.—Gaseous distension of the intestine.

I T remains for us to examine the etiological conditions which, while being compatible with the practice of singing, are susceptible of impeding the play of the muscles of respiration, and of injuring the functional activity of the lungs. We shall not speak of those acute or chronic affections, local or general, which profoundly affect the organism, and in the course of which we can no longer dream of the least vocal exercise. We shall confine ourselves to indicating certain conditions of disease and of overwork, which occasion a

diminution of the vital capacity often unknown to the singer himself. We may remark
how important it is for the singer to know his
normal spirometric measurement, and how
much information he could thus give the
physician, who would then be enabled to
immediately appreciate slight respiratory
deficiency ; for it is not possible to determine
offhand the maximum quantity of air that
an individual in full health ought to expire.
Tables for this purpose, based upon the
height of the individual, the sex, the muscular
force, the height of the trunk, the body weight,
the diameter of the chest, lead to valuations
which are at best but little exact. Experiments repeated upon a great number of
healthy persons have shown us that in many
cases the famous laws of Hutchinson cannot
be applied to figures volumetrically ascer-
tained. We have also formed the habit of
not affirming any volumetric diminution in
any disease before we have been assured of
the veritable pulmonary capacity in the normal
capacity, by direct and ulterior researches,
which would have been rendered unnecessary
had the singer been in possession of his
spirometric measurements.

Fatigue of the thoracic muscles is a pretty constant cause of expiratory feebleness. It is easy to understand how the muscular agents, overtaxed in consequence of exaggeration in the duration of the exercise, or the emission of notes produced with too great intensity, will become less apt to furnish the sum of the work, which is exacted by the large movements of thoracic amplification and retraction. All professors of singing have met with cases of this kind. All specialists have observed laryngeal affections in pupils, who have experienced malaise, weight, trembling, painful spots in the region of the ribs, amongst *debutants* who have already experienced slight respiratory impediment, or a little difficulty in holding sounds. If the spirometer be used then, it will be immediately seen, when respiration has become normal again, that there has been a lowering of the vital capacity. We have already said that Mandl considered this overtaxing of the thoracic muscles to be one of the ordinary consequences of the use of the clavicular type of breathing. It is possible if there has been abuse or excess on the part of the singer ; but otherwise the judicious and moderate employment of this or that type cannot create alone a condition of respiratory and laryngeal feebleness.

On the contrary, it is sometimes hurtful to change the type of respiration which the singer has employed for a long time.

Let us suppose the case of a singer habituated to the costal method of breathing, which permits him to obtain 4,500 cubic centimètres of air, and who may be compelled by a professor to adopt the abdominal type, with which he can introduce into his lungs only 4,000 cubic centimètres of air. The artist has half a litre of air the less at his disposal, or, as he is not always conscious of this loss and still seeks to obtain the same vocal effects, he must compensate the feebleness of his wind power by increase of laryngeal strength, which will lead to the affections of the vocal cords already mentioned.

A diminution of the functional activity of the lungs may result from a nasal affection ; that is a fact which we have demonstrated with the spirometer, by noting the feeble lowerings of the volume of air in certain individuals simply presenting a slight alteration of the pituitary membrane.*

* *Récherches spirométriques.* 1890.

Dating from a long time clinicians, Dupuytren, Shaw, Chassaignac, and Lambron among others, have been struck with the peculiar configuration which the thorax presents in subjects respiring through the mouth.

"The chest," said Robert,* "instead of being of regular and rounded surface over its lateral regions, is, on the contrary, depressed, flat, and sometimes concave, as if, at the period when the ribs are still soft and flexible, they had been compressed one side towards the other."

But these observers, not suspecting the existence of the pharyngeal tonsil, attributed these conditions of the thorax to hypertrophy of the palatine tonsils. It is well known to-day that these costal malformations are met with especially in individuals who have their nasal passages obstructed by adenoid vegetations. These subjects breathe entirely through the mouth, at least during sleep, when the arch of the palate falls inert upon the base of the tongue, thus presenting a new obstacle to the entry of air. There is then insufficiency of the inspiratory current, with panting and breathlessness during the

* *Bulletin thérapeutique.* 1843.

day upon the least effort, and frequent wakings, nightmares, and even profuse sweats, during the night.

We may easily conceive that these affections of respiration are not due exclusively to the presence of adenoid vegetations in the naso-pharynx, but may equally well be engendered by any affection which determines impermeability of the nasal fossæ, such as hypertrophic catarrh, mucous polypi, deviations, spurs of the septum, foreign bodies, etc.

Over and above these symptoms, of a purely mechanical order, disorders of the nose are capable of provoking another series of phenomena, of reflex character, in the chest. We refer to those dyspnœic affections which are well known to-day, and which we studied in 1882.*

A true erectile tissue is contained in the pituitary membrane. These cavernous bodies, with small meshes, superficial, and with lacunæ which are pretty large in its deepest parts, are contained in the inferior turbinated, the edge of the middle turbinated, and the posterior extremities of the turbinated bodies,

* *Sur les rapports de l'asthme et des polypes muqueux du nez.* 1882.

They also exist over the septum. This tissue is made turgescent by the slightest and most variable causes ; the terminal fibres of the trigeminal nerve are excited, and in certain individuals this irritation produces different reflexes, which may be manifested in distant regions of the organism. Amongst these, bronchial spasm deserves to be mentioned as of the greatest importance, and there are now but few physicians who do not admit the nasal origin of certain asthmas. Facts as numerous as demonstrative have been recorded in support of this.

To those pathological proofs establishing the important *rôle* which nasal affections play in the production of certain dyspnœas, we may add the facts furnished by experiments on animals. François Frank* operating upon dogs, cats, and rabbits, in which the nasal vault had been previously laid bare, and the turbinated and external wall of one side had been removed, found that suffocative bronchial spasm, energetic enough to be recognised by depression of the intercostal spaces in the tracheotomised animals, could be obtained by

* *Archives de physiologie normale et pathologique.* 1889.

every lively stimulation of the nose over the turbinateds, especially when the mucous membrane was inflamed. Thus, from nasal irritation giving rise to a reflex, or in consequence of deficient nasal permeability, affections of the respiratory function of variable intensity may arise. Sometimes the disorders produced constitute formidable crises of oppression, or are manifested by thoracic malformations. In other cases, on the contrary, the modifications of the regular play of the respiratory functions are scarcely sensible, no true dyspnœa is occasioned, and they are scarcely indicated except by the spirometer or pneumographic instruments.

These slight diminutions of the pulmonary capacity ought always to be sought for in singers affected either with hypertrophic rhinitis or naso-pharyngeal catarrh, and who complain of a certain difficulty in holding sounds or emitting acute notes. We cure the alterations of the voice by appropriate treatment of the nasal affection which has caused the trouble by lowering the respiratory power.

We may quote the case of a young artist possessing a superb soprano voice, well toned, flexible, and extensive, reaching from ut^3 to *re⁵*. In 1885 this individual noticed that her voice was no longer so firm as before ; if she sang for long she felt discomfort and heat in the larynx; respiration was less ample than before ; there was general lassitude, and painful sensations in the thorax were felt after long exercises ; there was a neurotic condition, irritability, and tendency to weep. There was no breathlessness during walking. The spirometric volume was 2,900 cubic centimètres.

There was nothing abnormal in the larynx, pharynx, or chest, but there was a double hypertrophic rhinitis, especially on the left side, where there was a deviation of the septum and a cartilaginous spur. We proposed to the patient rhino-surgical treatment, but our advice was not followed.

In 1886 the vocal troubles were accentuated, the patient could no longer reach the *ut³* and the *re⁵*. There was appreciable tremor, a difficulty in producing *mezza di voce*, and vocalisation was defective. There were, moreover, frequent attacks of hoarseness after vocal effort, and without taking chills, or any external cause. During one of these attacks the laryngeal mucous membrane and the inferior vocal cords were the seat of a lively redness. Moreover, the patient had lost her wind, and thoracic fatigue was more pronounced. The spirometer registered 2,700 cubic centimètres.

The cartilaginous spur of the septum was resected; and the hypertrophic rhinitis was treated with the galvano-cautery. Absolute rest of the larynx was enjoined for eight months. In 1887, a year after operation, the pulmonary capacity was 3,400 cubic centimètres : there were no more attacks of hoarseness, and the voice was partly restored. At the end of 1888 this artist told us that she sang as well as before, and had achieved a number of brilliant successes both in France and abroad.

We might relate other cases of the same kind, but it is useless to reproduce them, since they are nearly the same as the case described. The respiratory reflex arising from a hypertrophic rhinitis or mucous polypi is ordinarily developed in subjects of the class of arthritic neuropaths—that is to say, individuals attainted with neurotic temperament and presenting besides the attributes of the gouty or rheumatic diathesis.

These patients, often born of asthmatic parents, are themselves likely subjects for asthma. The predisposition being already there, or acquired, it is sufficient, in order to provoke spasmodic phenomena, to have some determining cause, such as an irritation, which is not always seated in the nose. The palatine tonsils, the pharyngeal wall, the lingual tonsil, the stomach, the skin, and the ovaries, are foci of excitation. Whatever may be the origin of the impression which reaches the medulla oblongata, and is reflected to the bronchial filaments of the pneumogastric, the respiratory trouble could not take the dyspnœic form and consist simply of a diminution of vital capacity, which it would be useful in artistes to determine by the spirometer.

Pulmonary emphysema is an affection to which singers are particularly exposed, as also are all individuals whose professions necessitate powerful and repeated efforts, such as porters, labourers, commissionaires, public criers, players of wind instruments, glass blowers, etc. This pathological condition is characterised by the formation in the lungs of ampullary cavities which result from the dilatation and fusion of alveoli, the walls of which have been altered by nutritive changes. These thin, atrophied walls fail in resistance, and, becoming distended, are ruptured by expiratory pressures which would be insufficient to overcome the elasticity of a normal lung ; and the more frequently use is made of high pressures, as in the act of singing, the more is the development of the disorder favoured.

When emphysema has affected a large area of the pulmonary organ it gives rise to a group of symptoms which render its diagnosis easy. Such patients have short and noisy respiration, are breathless at the least movement, they walk with short steps, speaking obliges them to cut short their phrases, in order to take breath, they cannot lie in the horizontal position, and at nights are obliged to sit upright in bed.

The configuration of the thorax assumes in these patients a special character ; the chest becomes round, barrel-shaped, the intercostal spaces are enlarged, the sternum pushed forwards, depressions are seen in the clavicular regions. Percussion gives a resonant note, more striking than in the normal chest, the vocal vibrations are enfeebled to palpitation,

and there is a notable diminution of the vesi-
cular murmur in auscultation; respiration
takes a rough tone, inspiration is difficult and
expiration prolonged. Generally, sonorous
and sibilant or moist *râles* are perceived, signs
of the bronchial catarrh which usually accom-
panies emphysema, and is the cause of the
spasmodic cough and muco-purulent expectoration of which these patients complain. The
spirometer shows that when the affection has
reached thus far, the vital capacity of the
lungs has diminished in the enormous proportions of 40 to 60 per cent. ; and according to
Wintrich the volume of expired air falls from
4,000 cubic centimètres to 2,000, or even less.

All vocal exercises have for long been
abandoned when the respiratory capacity has
submitted to such a reduction, and unhappily
no therapeutic means can then restore to the
lungs their power and elasticity.

On the contrary, under well-directed treatment, based on the administration of iodide of
potassium internally, and the employment of
compressed air, a winter residence at the
Mediterranean, and a summer sojourn at
mineral springs, we have a chance of arresting
the march of emphysema, if it is not yet too

advanced. The curative results will be more pronounced the earlier the disease is treated. But it is almost impossible to recognise the time when the disease appears first, the objective symptoms only being appreciable when a great number of pulmonary alveoli are already dilated.

However, before the appearance of any other signs, even before there is the least breathlessness, the singer experiences difficulty in holding sounds, and giving them the intensity he used to do, or in singing musical phrases as long as formerly. He feels that his wind fails him. If the spirometric diminution is consecutive to an acute bronchitis, or an attack of asthma, and if the examination of the chest and other organs reveals nothing abnormal, the physician ought to suspect emphysema, and act accordingly.

Writers have drawn attention to the diminution of the vital capacity observed at the commencement of pulmonary tuberculosis, and Lasègue especially has insisted upon the service rendered by the spirometer in diagnosis, which is sometimes so difficult.

Certain congestive conditions localised at the base of the lungs, especially in arthritic subjects, determine only a short, dry cough and slight respiratory trouble.

Contusions of the costal region, muscular pains of rheumatic nature, may limit the movements of the thorax. Respiratory troubles of a mechanical order will also be the only symptoms perceived by the patient in certain latent forms of pleurisy without fever or pain.

Lastly, the movements of the diaphragm are impeded by certain affections of the stomach, such as gastralgia and flatulent dyspepsia ; the gaseous distensions of the intestine so frequently observed in nervous persons, accumulations in the colon, utero-ovarian disorders, will have the same effect, and will deprive the artist of a portion of the respiratory power.

APPENDIX.

[*Note to p.* 104.]

THE RESONANCE OF THE THORAX.

IN their paper in the *Journal of Physiology*, vol. xi., 1890, Sewall and Pollard write: "The power and quality of a voice depend not so much on the mere trembling of the vocal reeds, as on the sympathetic vibration of the air in the resonance chambers above and below the larynx. . . . Helmholtz clearly demonstrated that the difference in quality of tones having the same pitch depends upon the nature and relative power of the various upper partials which accompany the fundamental in every musical tone." This has been generally admitted as regards the upper respiratory channel—nose, mouth, naso-pharynx, and parts above the larynx—the different forms and sizes of which cavities must produce differences of quality of tones emitted through the larynx; but, as Sewall and Pollard point out, "comparatively little attention has been paid to the function of the thorax as a resonance chamber. . . . It is generally admitted that the chest, by virtue of the condensation of air within it during phonation, responds with more powerful resonance to the sounds emitted by the larynx than do the cavities above that organ. . . . From physical considerations we should expect that the perfection of resonance in the chest would vary with the tension of the bounding walls, and that its fundamental note and overtones would be altered by change in size and shape of the cavity, with the accompanying variation in the contained air-channel. The results of experiments undertaken with a view of testing this point respond decidedly in the affirmative. By their experiments, Sewall and Pollard conclude that with a decrease in its vertical, and increase in its transverse, diameters, "the chest cavity so changes in its resonant properties that its fundamental note is elevated, while with diminution of its transverse section and increase of the vertical dimension, the proper note of the chamber is lowered."

The best effect for vocalisation and for the physiological needs of the organism as requiring much less exertion for the production and maintenance of any given note, will be attained when the sympathetic vibration of air in the lungs most nearly harmonises with that of the vocal cords.

These experiments lead to the inevitable conclusion that the best effects are obtained by the harmonious working of the whole of the muscular system of the respiratory function, and not by the confining of the act to the intervention of one group of muscles, or in attempting a purely diaphragmatic system of respiration.

Note to p. 154.]

THE INFLUENCE OF ODOURS AND PERFUMES UPON THE
VOICE.

IT has long been known that the inhalation of the
odours arising from certain plants or animals may in
certain individuals produce the most curious effects,
and though doubtless some of the cases recorded in
older times have about them a somewhat apochryphal
air—such as that recorded by Cloquet of a lady found
dead in bed, whose demise was attributed to the emanations from lilies, which she had preserved in her bed-
room ; the case of the death of a bishop from the odour of
roses, recorded by Cromer ; and other similar cases of
ancient medical history—there is no doubt a solid
substratum of truth in the popular objection to keeping
flowers in the sleeping apartment. The ill effects are,
however, doubtless due to the respiration of carbonic
acid gas in confined spaces. The reader in search of
the curious will find gratification in the perusal of the
very learned and scientific essays of Dr. John Mackenzie,
of Baltimore ("Rose Cold," *Am. Journ. of the Med.
Sciences*, 1886, etc.) That the odours of certain flowers
may produce asthma has been recognised for long—
indeed, ever since Van Helmont in 1682 published
the fact that asthma, migraine, syncope, or palpitation,
might be thus caused. Most people are familiar with
the fact that the sight of, or emanations from certain
animals, *e.g.*, cats, may, in some curiously-constituted
individuals, produce an attack of asthma.

The Americans have an affection which is known in that country as " Rose Cold," *i.e.*, a coryza, which is attributed to the odour of these flowers.

Closely related to these conditions is " Hay Fever," which some medical writers (Hack, Joal) have regarded as being as much due to the stimulation of the olfactory nerve by certain perfumes, as to direct irritation by pollen, as is generally believed, in this country at least. It would be out of place here to deal further with these matters, the object of this note being to call attention to a communication lately made by Dr. Joal to the *Revue Mensuelle de Laryngologie* (1894, Nos. 3 and 5) upon the influence of certain odours upon the singing voice, a subject which he properly remarks has not received the attention it should have done among medical men, although singers themselves are not unaware of the pernicious effects of certain flowers, *e.g.*, the rose, the violet, the tuberose, the lily, the gardenia, heliotrope, etc., upon the organs of phonation. It thus becomes a subject, not merely of curiosity, but of importance to the singer. Dr. Joal thus sums up his conclusions :—

1. In addition to the symptoms indicated by various writers, viz., migraine, vertigo, syncope, spasms, convulsions, nausea, vomiting, palpitation, cardialgia, etc., odours may provoke alterations in the voice.

2. These disorders may occur in different parts of the organ—the resonating, the vibrating, or the motor element.

3. The olfactory impression gives rise to a reflex action, which determines turgescence of the erectile tissue of the nose, and excitation of

the filaments of the tirgeminal nerve, whence
is superadded a secondary reflex, determining
vasomotor affections of the nasal mucous membrane (pharyngitis and laryngitis by propagation);
vasomotor affections of the laryngeal mucous
membrane (secondary paralysis of the constric-
tor muscles); nervous cough (secondary vocal
congestion); spasms of the bronchial muscles.

4. These reflex conditions may modify the "timbre"
of the voice, rendering high notes less easy of
production, or less limpid; or may produce
hoarseness, or even aphonia; or, by diminishing
the respiratory power, may lessen the intensity,
volume, or duration, of sounds, or rapidly impair
the powers of the singer.

5. These alterations occur by preference in persons
of nervous temperament, with excessive sensibility, and especially in arthritic neuropathic
individuals predisposition is created by any
hypertrophic lesion of the nasal mucous membrane.

6. The employment of cocaine as an intra-nasal
application, either by swabbing, spray, or pow-
der, will be profitable to subjects thus affected.

The facts which Dr. Joal states are incontestable, and
his explanation of them is physiologically correct. If
we may take exception to any of his views it is only as
to the method of treatment of these cases. Cocaine is
one of the most pernicious drugs a singer can employ.
It is a most dangerous drug for any one to use except
under strict medical supervision. And this much is said
to warn non-medical readers of this work against its

employment. To the professional reader it may be remarked that the best treatment of such largely psychological cases must be first to remove the offending cause, viz., the exposure to emanations from powerfully-smelling flowers; secondly, to correct such hypertrophies of the nasal mucous membrane as already exist, by appropriate surgical treatment; and lastly, but chiefly, to endeavour to brace up the nervous system by the administration of nervine tonics and proper treatment, which need scarcely be further indicated.

A singer should always remember that in playing with cocaine, however pleasant the temporary relief may be, he is playing with fire. It is a drug which has been so commonly used, without proper medical advice, that it is necessary to give this emphatic warning against its employment.

[*Note to page* 182.]

LARYNGITIS IN SINGERS.

As Moure, of Bordeaux, has pointed out, it is to the sopranos that the greatest integrity of the vocal cords is most essential, next baritones and mezza sopranos, finally basses and contraltos, who may sing with unimpaired effect when the larynx is distinctly catarrhal. While it is quite possible for a soprano to go through a long performance with congested vocal cords, with little, if any, impairment of effect, it is a practice to be condemned. We are frequently consulted by a singer suffering from an attack of sub-acute laryngitis, who desires to be pulled through some special effort. It must be recollected that it is at best but a dangerous experiment, and one which may lead to the enforcement of complete rest and prolonged treatment subsequently. In such conditions, Solis Cohen recommends the administration of a sharp emetic, the patient then being directed to rest until the time of the performance, sucking ice, and keeping a cold compress over the neck. In the intervals of the play the singer may inhale tincture of benzoin. Quinine (1 grain with ¼ grain of nux vomica) every two hours, with coca wine and faradaism externally to the neck, is recommended by Sajous. We have pulled a singer through a fine performance by treating the congested larynx with sprays of chloride of zinc frequently applied during the day, and inhalations of benzoin during the performance; but instances in which this treatment should be adopted for a singer with sub-acute congestion of the larynx should be very exceptional, and only undertaken under urgent circumstances. The singer would do far better to defer the performance.

[*Note to page* 183, *et seq.*]

LOCAL CONDITIONS LEADING TO IMPAIRMENT OF
THE VOICE.

DR. HOLBROOK CURTIS, of New York, has recently published a very interesting paper, " The Effects on the Vocal Cords of Improper Methods of Singing " (*New York Medical Journal*, Jan. 20th, 1894), and as to which he gave a further demonstration at the British Laryngological Association meeting, July, 1894. Many singers are subject to minute papillomata and fibromata upon their vocal cords, striations and congestions of the vocal cords, or nodules on their free edges, such conditions having been observed in persons who, in singing, make use of the *coup de glotte*, and are trained with daily exercises upon the single vowels "o" and "A." This *coup de glotte* ("stroke of the glottis") cannot be made without bringing the vocal cords in contact, producing by attrition the nodules so often seen between the middle and anterior third of the cords.

The cure for these conditions, is, according to Curtis, not the curette, forceps, or cautery, but exercising the intrinsic muscles of the larynx, which causes tension of the cords. This is obtained by tones made *dans le masque*, or focussed in the face, the breathing being inferior costal, or diaphragmatic, the upper ribs raised, and the chin depressed almost to the sternum, the trachea being drawn downwards, and the thyroid depressed. The word "mau" (or "ma") is used, the M tone being made with the mouth, which is at first closed, so as to obtain complete relaxation of all the pharyngeal muscles, and the tone is allowed to break upon the lips as loudly as possible, without the contraction of a single muscle in the neck or pharynx. The theory is that under these conditions the cords are in the greatest possible state of tension. They vibrate without a point of contact, and the membrane receives a kind of massage. Curtis maintains that this exercise has restored, in a few days, cords supposed to have been permanently injured by singers' nodes, and that this method of vocal gymnastics is productive of great strength and brilliancy of tone, the constant practice of it doing away entirely with the fatigue produced by overwork, and so-called relaxation of the cords. (See *Journal of Laryngology*, August 1894, p. 495.)

It would seem scarcely necessary to impress upon singers the necessity of having adenoid vegetations, enlarged palatine tonsils, or lingual adenoids, nasal obstructions, and granular pharyngitis, operated upon, were it not that a prejudice exists sometimes against operative interference. It is a mistake to imagine that such conditions ever "disappear of themselves," and the correction of such local conditions is imperative, so as to procure proper breathing through the nose, greater resonance in the upper air-passages, and to prevent the faulty production of voice, and fatigue of muscles, which will surely follow, quite apart from the constant tendency to catarrhs of the naso-pharyngeal and laryngeal passages, which constantly recur in such conditions. Singers sometimes date some alteration in their voice from slight operative interference, which, however, is erroneous.

COCAINE.

WE have before remarked that this is a drug the employment of which to the larynx of a singer is most pernicious. Dr. John Mackenzie has made a remark in which we cannot but agree, that to use cocaine to

the larynx of a singer about to go on the stage is
" second only to hanging." We have known of a voice
impaired for years by the well-meant, but injudicious
use of cocaine to the larynx. The use of cocaine
lozenges so frequently employed is not to be recommended. Relaxation of the vocal cords, and even
paresis, follow in some cases, and the voice is
rendered deficient in tone and brilliancy.

THE END.

Printed by Hazell, Watson, & Viney, Ld., London and Aylesbury.

www.ingramcontent.com/pod-product-compliance
Lightning Source LLC
Chambersburg PA
CBHW030315270326
41926CB00010B/1372